NRCME
STUDY GUIDE

by

David A. Thorpe, DC, DACBOH

Certified Medical Examiner
National Trainer for the "Accredited DOT Training Program"

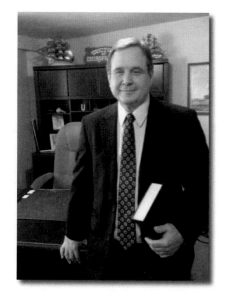

Dr. David Thorpe is the President and owner of WorkRite Safety, an occupational consulting company located in Upstate New York. He has served in many State and National organizations representing his profession, and specialty, and has worked with the National Registry in its development and implementation. He is also one of a handful of national trainers for an accredited training program necessary to sit for the examination.

In addition to being the author of this study guide he also has authored "The CME's Guide to the DOT Physical Exam", the most current and up to date manual available on the market today. It is a clinical reference manual and business guide for those who wish to work in this area of specialty within occupational medicine. It is a "living manual", meaning that updates to the manual may be purchased for a nominal fee so that it will always remain current with all regulations and guidelines. These updates are made available once or twice per year through the website (www.cmedot.com), and you will also receive a quarterly newsletter providing timely information concerning changes in policy, new regulations, upcoming training, best practice decisions and more. For those purchasing the manual through Amazon or another outlet other than the website you may contact us via the email listed on the website so that we can include you with all of the above benefits.

The manual is organized as a table-top reference manual which is portable and can be used both within the provider's facility, but also at remote locations. The examiner will be able to reference conditions, medications and regulatory information within seconds. It contains not only all regulatory and guidance information, but also a quick reference for disqualifying and modifying medications, contact information for Federal agencies, all State DMV's, professional organizations, a section relating to the business of drug and alcohol testing, marketing your services and much more. To purchase the manual, or any of the other products necessary to successfully working with the trucking industry, you may log onto www.cmedot.com.

HOW TO USE YOUR NRCME STUDY GUIDE

This study guide was prepared so that all defined categories identified by the National Registry as being critical to the Certified Medical Examiner and specifically identified as areas to be tested, are organized separately and contain regulatory and advisory guidance for specifically defined conditions, their treatment, required testing, and defined physical examination criteria. Additionally, each section and its components provide page reference to **"The CME's Guide to the DOT Physical Exam"** so that the candidate may expand on their understanding of each category or condition.

The separate categories are organized as follows:

1. The Healthy Driver Physical and Certification
2. Regulations to remember
3. Documentation
4. Certification Periods
5. Waiting Periods
6. Required Medical Clearance
7. Required and Recommended Testing
8. Counseling Requirements
9. Waivers, Exemptions and SPE
10. Disqualifying Conditions (Temporary and Permanent)
11. Disqualifying Medications and Medications of Concern
12. NRCME Practice Test

It is recommended that each candidate first study and become knowledgeable with each category above, reference the CME Guide and their class notes from training prior to taking the practice test.

When taking the practice test, I would also recommend you set a timer for 120 minutes (allowing about 1 minute per question which equals the time allowed in the actual test), so that you can also develop a pace for the test. Once completed, then refer to the answers at the end of the booklet, and not before. You will develop an understanding of areas of strengths and weaknesses as you continue your preparation. A score of 75 should be a good indication that you are ready to take the test.

Good Luck!
Dr. David Thorpe

NRCME STUDY GUIDE

The Healthy Driver Physical and Certification

1. There are 8 parts to the DOT Physical Exam (2-1:2)
    A. Driver's Information
    B. Health History
    C. Vision
    D. Hearing
    E. Blood Pressure/Pulse
    F. Laboratory and other testing
    G. Physical Examination
    H. Certification Status
2. Required Components of all exams include
    A. Vision
    B. Hearing
    C. Blood Pressure/Pulse
    D. UA (if on dialysis, obtain this information from the treating provider)
3. Who can sign the examination form? (3-1:2)
    A. The Medical Examiner (CME)
    B. Optometrist
    C. Ophthalmologist
4. A discussion on discretionary and non discretionary standards (Best Practices)
    A. There are 13 standards overall. A non-discretionary standard indicates that you MUST follow the regulation or guideline and may not vary from this. Non-discretionary standards are:
        i.   Vision – The driver must be 20/40 in both eyes and in each eye independently. They must also have 70 degrees of peripheral vision and be able to distinguish signal red, green and amber (yellow). If they do not meet the above criteria they may apply for a vision exemption. The CME must provide a copy of the certificate and long form marked "Accompanied by a _____ waiver/ exemption. The driver must present the exemption at the time of certification. They may also use glasses or contacts, and if so, the medical examiner must mark this in the certification section on the card and the long form. (1-1:5, 3-1:1, 3-1:2, 3-1:3)
        ii. Hearing – The driver must pass the whisper test, or audiometric test (with an average hearing loss of less than or equal to 40 db measured at 500 Hz, 1000 Hz and 2000 Hz). If they use a hearing aide, you must mark this in the certification section of the card and long form, as well as the corresponding section within the exam itself. If they do not meet the above criteria, they may apply for a hearing exemption. The CME must provide a copy of the certificate and long form marked "Accompanied by a _____ waiver/ exemption. (1-1:6, 2-1:4, 3-1:3, 3-1:4)

The examiner is required to observe the tympanic membrane on every examination.

    iii. Epilepsy – The FMCSA definition of epilepsy is 2 events, or the use of anti-seizure medication. Always DQ the driver with a clinical diagnosis of epilepsy. See Disqualifying conditions and medications, along with waiting periods. If the driver suffers from epilepsy or has a seizure disorder from an unknown cause (controlled or uncontrolled), they may apply for a seizure exemption. The CME must provide them with a copy of the certificate and long form marked "Accompanied by a _____ waiver/exemption. (1-1:5, 2-1:9, 2-1:14, 7-1:11, appendix).

    iv. Blood Pressure – Follow guidance regarding Stage 1, 2 or 3. Once diagnosed, they will always have a shortened certification time, usually 1 year, whether they are treated or not. They may treat with mediations or by exercise and diet. See section for Certification time frames and disqualifying conditions. (1-1:25, 3-1:5).

5. A comment about taking a History. (2-1:2, 2-1:3)

    A. In taking a history always remember that the driver must first fill out their section (driver information and history) in total, and sign and date the form. Realize however that the driver frequently marks the form incorrectly, sometimes intentionally but usually due to a lack of understanding or simply not taking the time to read each question. Therefore, as you review the history you should ask the driver the following questions.

"Are you currently taking any prescriptive or OTC medications, vitamins or minerals? Have you ever been hospitalized, had a serious illness or had surgeries in your lifetime (although the form lists the past 5 years, you need to query the driver as to injuries and illnesses throughout his life in case they may effect your decision)? Have you suffered any head injuries, had seizures? Do you have any eye disorders or conditions, such as cataracts, glaucoma, macular degeneration, or loss of a lens? Have you had any ear problems, loss of hearing and do you wear a hearing aide? Do you have any heart problems such as having a pace maker or ICD, valvular problems or suffered a heart attack? Do you or have you ever been treated for high blood pressure? Do you have any lung problems such as shortness of breath, asthma, COPD or emphysema? Do you suffer any digestive disorders? Do you or have you been treated for anxiety, depression, PTSD, ADHD or any other mental disorder? Have you ever fainted or lost consciousness? Have you ever suffered from dizzy spells? Do you or have you ever been treated for any sleep disorders, such as narcolepsy, or sleep apnea? Do you snore loudly, or suffer from daytime sleepiness? Have you ever suffered a stroke, TIA or any paralysis? Do you have all of your fingers and toes (of course you will notice any variation from this during your exam)? Do you suffer from any spinal disease, have chronic back problems or have any limitations attached to you from injuries that would limit your ability to lift, reach, sit climb, control an oversized wheel, shift gears, load and unload a trailer etc.? Have you ever been treated for alcohol or drug abuse? Finally you should ask if the driver is a smoker or non-smoker and record this in the comments section of the history in the long form.

Note: For the driver who has a benign history and normal examination the maximum certification will always be 2 years.

Regulations to remember

1. 49 CFR 391.41 – Physical Qualifications for Drivers (1-1:4)
    A. (b)(1) – Loss of Limb (7-1:6)
    B. (b)(2) – Limb Impairment (7-1:6)
    C. (b)(3) – Diabetes (1-1:5, 1-1:20, 1-1:26, 2-1:5, 2-1:6)
    D. (b)(4) - Cardiovascular Conditions (1-1:5, 5-1:1 through 5-1:32)
    E. (b)(5) – Respiratory Dysfunction (1-1:5, 5-2:1 through 5-2:25)
    F. (b)(6) – Hypertension (1-1:5, 1-1:25, 3-1:5)
    G. (b)(7) – Rheumatic, Arthritic, Orthopedic, Muscular, Neuromuscular or Vascular disease (1-1:5, 7-1:1 though 7-1:14)
    H. (b)(8) – Epilepsy (1-1:5, 2-1:9, 2-1:14, 7-1:11, appendix)
    I. (b)(9) – Mental Disorders (1-1:5, 2-1:10)
    J. (b)(10) – Vision (1-1:5, 1-1:20, 1-1:24, 3-1:2, 3-1:3)
        i. (b)(11) – Hearing (1-1:6, 2-1:4, 3-1:3, 3-1:4)
        ii. (b)(12) – Drug Use (1-1:6, 9-1:2, 9-1:9, 9-1:14, 9-1:21)
        iii. (b)(13) – Alcoholism (1-1:6, 7-1:9, 7-1:11, 9-1:2, 9-1:16, 9-1:18, 9-1:19, 9-1:28)
2. 49 CFR 391.45 – Persons who must be medically examined and certified (1- 1:6)
3. 49 CFR 391.47 – Resolution of conflicts (1-1:7)
4. 49 CFR 391.49 – Alternative physical qualifications for loss or impairment of limbs (SPE) (1-1:4, 1-1:9, 1-1:16, 7-1:6)
5. 49 CFR 391.62 – Limited exemptions for intra-city zone drivers (1-1:18)
6. 49 CFR 391.64 – Grand-fathering for vision and diabetic Waiver program (1-1:20)
7. 49 CFR 391.43 – The Role of the Medical Examiner
8. A comment about regulations vs. guidelines
    A. Regulations are enacted by law and take time and effort to enact. Consequently there are fewer regulations, and most of the guidance provided by the FMCSA is in the form of guidelines.
    B. Guidelines are just that…they are intended that you follow, but you may have some leeway in the decision making process. In essence, you better have a good reason for varying from a guideline.
    C. "Best Practice" decisions are made when there is no specific guideline or regulation to follow. You must, based on your history and examination, determine if the driver is medically qualified to drive a CMV.
        i. 1% rule – This applies in the decision making process. If there is in the examiners opinion, greater than a 1% chance in the next year of a sudden incapacitation, you must DQ the driver.
        ii. In making a decision for medical certification consider:

          1. The condition

          2. Its treatment

          3. The episodic nature of the condition

Documentation (1-1:23, 2-1:3)

1. The history must be thoroughly documented, including:
   - A. Date of onset
   - B. Diagnosis
   - C. Treating physician name, address and phone number if available
   - D. Any current limitations
   - E. Current medications (including OTC), nutritional supplements, herbals etc.
2. Examination findings must be documented in the space provided.

In documenting information and findings, tag any yes answer in the history with a written number, and connect that number with the same written number in the comments section for the examiner. For any abnormalities identified in the examination section, utilize each numbered section, and repeat that number in the comments section for the examiner with a list of findings. Lastly, in the comments section of the examination, you should always include the driver's BMI (Body Mass Index) (4-1:1, 5-2:19).

Any correspondence from treating providers needs to be documented and attached.

          1. Its treatment

          2. Progression, remission and monitoring

Certification Periods

1. The following certification periods are defined by guidelines and regulations.
   - A. Benign history, negative exam – 2 years
   - B. Diabetes – non-insulin dependent – 1 year (2-1:6)
   - C. Diabetes – with insulin (diabetic) exemption or waiver – 1 year (2-1:6)
   - D. Hearing exemption – 1 year (3-1:4)
   - E. Epilepsy/seizure exemption – 1 year (2-1:10)
   - F. Other endocrine disorders – 2 years (2-1:7 through 2-1:10)
   - G. Mental disorders – if able to certify, maximum 1 year during treatment. Some disqualifying conditions and medications used to treat mental disorders. See those sections. (2-1:10 through 2-1:16)
   - H. Vision exemption – Certified for 1 year only. (3-1:3)
   - I. Blood Pressure – Anyone who has a history of Htn (treated with medication, diet or weight loss and exercise), and their blood pressure is below 140/90 at the time of the examination, may be granted a 1 year certificate unless they have a history of Stage 3 Htn, then the maximum certification period is for 6 months only. These certification periods will remain in effect for the rest of the drivers career. (3-1:5, 3-1:6).

Guidance is somewhat complicated due to recent changes in the regulations, and with confusion resultant from the errors in the long form and 49 CFR 391.41.

    i. Stage 1 (140-159/90-99) – If this is the first time diagnosed (confirmed by 2 readings taken on the same day), you may grant them a 1-year certificate. If they have a history of Htn, such as a previous reading on another exam (you will notice they have a 1 year card already, or they are currently taking Htn medications for example), then they only receive a 1-time 3 month certificate. Within the 3 months, they must have a BP reading from a provider (can be their PCP for example, or may be the CME), < or = 140/90. You would date the certification card for the original date of the examination. If they do not lower their BP < or = 140/90 within the 3-month time frame, they will be disqualified. Furthermore, if it is greater than 3 months before they lower their BP to an acceptable level, they should undergo another examination.

    ii. Stage 2 (160-179/100-109) – They are granted a 1-time 3- month certificate and follow the requirements for Stage 1 as listed above. The maximum certification will be for 1 year.

    iii. Stage 3 (180 or above/110 or above) – They are automatically DQ'd, until their BP is < or = 140/90. Their maximum certification will be for 6 months for the rest of the driver's career.

    iv. If the driver were to improve their health situation by loosing weight, exercise etc., and were taken off of their hypertensive medication, and it remained stable for a period of 2 years, the CME may choose to provide the driver with a 2 year certificate.

J. All certifiable cardiac conditions (Ischemic heart disease, valvular heart disease, and congestive heart failure, cardiac arrhythmias including pace makers, congenital heart problems, peripheral vascular disease, including intermittent claudication that is asymptomatic at rest, DVT and pulmonary embolism, AAA, and those drivers with multiple coronary heart disease risk factors (modifiable and non modifiable) most will be certified for 1 year. (5-1:1 through 5-1:32). The exceptions are as follows:

    i. Heart transplant is certified for 6 months.

    ii. Some valvular conditions may be less than 1 year.

    iii. For PCI (angioplasty), the initial certification is for 3 to 6 months

In each category listed above, you will have to refer to waiting periods, required testing, medical clearance, and DQ medical conditions and medications.

K. Respiratory conditions are less regulated. For most you will be able to certify the driver for a period of 2 years. This includes infectious disease, non-infectious disease, allergies, post pneumonectomy/lung resection, trachestomy, primary and secondary lung carcinoma, lung transplants, all will be certifiable for 2 years. For OSA and DVT and Pulmonary thromboembolism, only certify for 1 year. (5-1:1 thorough 5-1:25)

In each category listed above, you will have to refer to waiting periods, required testing, medical clearance, and DQ medical conditions and medications.

L. All certifiable abdominal conditions, GU, GI, hematologic disorders, neoplastic disorders, and hernias may be certified for 2 years. (6-1:1 through 6-1:6)

In each category above, you will have to refer to disqualifying conditions, medical clearance sections.

M. Orthopedic/neurologic conditions that are certifiable may be certified for 2 years. Exceptions include (7-1:1 through 7-1:14)
   i. History of Embolic/Thrombotic Stroke who can certify – 1 year.
   ii. History of Intracerebral and Subarachnoid Hemorrhage who can certify – 1 year.
   iii. History of TIA who can certify – 1 year.
   iv. History of mild or moderate TBI who can certify – 1 year.
   v. Acute seizures – structural insult to brain who can certify – 1 year.

There are a significant number of neurologic conditions that will DQ the driver, or may have waiting periods, or required medical clearance. Refer to those sections for this information. Medications may also be problematic.

Waiting Periods

1. The following waiting periods are defined by the guidelines and regulations. Remember, if more than 1 waiting period is involved, the longer waiting period applies.
   A. Seizure disorder (1-1:5, 2-1:9, 2-1:14, 7-1:14)
      i. FMCSA definition of epilepsy is 2 or more events or use of anti seizure medication to control seizures (see section on DQ for epilepsy of seizure disorders).
      ii. If 1 event of unknown cause, and no anti seizure medication is required, the waiting period is 5 years (see section on required clearance).
      iii. If from a known cause (medication reaction, high fever for example), the waiting period is 0 to 6 months (Best Practice decision, see section on required medical clearance).
      iv. If the driver has met or exceeded 10 years with out the use of anti seizure medication (under medical direction) and has not suffered a seizure, they may be considered for medical certification (Best Practice). See also section on exemptions.
   B. Mental Disorders (2-1:10 through 2-1:16)
      i. Severe depression/thoughts of suicide or suicide attempt – 1 year
      ii. Non-psychotic major depression, no suicide attempt – 6 months.
      iii. Psychosis – symptom free for 1 year
         a. Brief episode of psychosis – 6 months
         b. Treatment involves the use of electroconvulsive therapy – 6 months

       iv. Cardiovascular disorders (5-1:1 through 5-1:32)
- a. Post MI – 2 months
- b. PCI (angioplasty) – 1 week
- c. Most surgical procedures except heart transplant – 3 months, except:
  - i. Heart transplant – 1 year
  - ii. Post-percutaneous balloon mitral valvotomy – 4 weeks.
  - iii. Surgical commissurotomy (valvular procedure) – 4 weeks.
  - iv. Post-balloon valvuloplasty – 1 month
  - v. Pacemaker for sinus node dysfunction, and AV block is 1 month, all other pacemakers are 3 months.
- d. Anticoagulation therapy – 1 month
  - i. Pulmonary embolism/Deep Vein Thrombosis (DVT) – 3 months

C. Respiratory disorders (5-2:1 through 5-2:25)
- i. OSA – 1 month CPAP, 3 months with surgery
  - a. The FMCSA definition of OSA is 30 hypo-apnea events per hour.
- ii. Use of Chantix for smoking, after discontinuing use – 2 weeks

D. Neurologic disorders (7-1:7 through 7-1:14)
- i. Thromboembolytic stroke – 1 year
- ii. Stroke involving medial or anterior cerebral artery – 5 years
- iii. Stroke with risk of seizures – 5 years
- iv. Transient Ischemic Attack (TIA) – 1 year
- v. Intracerebellar or subarachnoid hemorage
  - a. 1 year without risk of seizures
  - b. 5 years with risk of seizures.
- vi. Surgically repaired AV malformation or aneurysm with no seizure risk - 1 year
- vii. Surgically removed infratentorial meningiomas, acustic neuromas, pituitary adenomas, and benign spinal tumors – 2 years
- viii. Surgically removed supratentorial or spinal tumors – 2 years
- ix. Infections of the CNS
  - a. Viral encephalitis with early seizures – 10 years
  - b. Bacterial encephalitis with early seizures – 5 years
  - c. Infections of the CNS (bacterial meningitis, viral encephalitis without early seizures) – 1 year
- x. Traumatic Brain Injury (TBI)
  - a. Mild TBI without early seizures – 1 year
  - b. Mild TBI with early seizures – 2 years
  - c. Moderate TBI without early seizures – 2 years
  - d. Moderate TBI with early seizures – 5 years

xi. Benign Paroxysimal Vertigo and Vestibulopathy – 2 months

There are numerous variations in medical certification, waiting periods, required medical clearance, required testing, counseling, disqualifying medications and conditions etc. Please refer to these sections for this information.

Required Medical Clearance

1. A single episode of seizure resultant from a known cause (high fever, medication reaction etc.) – All (1-1:5, 2-1:9, 2-1:14, 7-1:11)
2. Mental disorders – All (2-1:10 through 2-1:16)
3. Drug and alcohol abuse – Any driver that admits to, is in treatment for   or is positive on a random drug or alcohol test, must have clearance from a "Substance Abuse Professional" (SAP) prior to being re-considered for driving. (1-1:6, 9-1:1 through 9-1:30)
4. Eye disorders - Best practice decision based on history and examination findings. Specific conditions such as Macular degeneration, glaucoma, cataracts, diabetic retinopathy and aphakia are mentioned in the regulation. Remember, an optometrist and/or ophthalmologist may sign the form (vision standard). (4-1:2 through 4-1:8)
5. Cardiac conditions – All (5-1:1 thorough 5-1:32)
6. Respiratory conditions – Assume for all chronic, not well controlled or   potentially incapacitation conditions (episodic nature and progression). This would be a "Best Practices" decision. Please refer also to section, dealing with required medical testing for those specific requirements which will also help your decision making process. (5-2:1 through 5-2:25).
7. Kidney, GU, GI, Hematologic, Neoplastic disorders – Best Practices. Clearance sought in all chronic and potentially incapacitating conditions. Consideration given to severity, progression and episodic nature, and treatment including side effects of medications. (6-1:1 through 6-1:6)
8. Orthopedic – Best practice decision with consultation recommended when there exists a current limitation or disability. (7-1:1 though 7-1:7)
9. Neurologic – Advised for all chronic and /or potentially progressive disease that is not disqualifying. Required for non-epileptic single episode seizure, cerebrovascular event, tumor, vascular malformation, infection of CNS and TBI. (7-1:7 through 7-1:14)

Required and Recommended Testing

1. Diabetes – A1c (Normal 4 to 6.5, a 10 however equates to 300 mb/dl which is low risk!). Any 10 or below would be certifiable. (2-1:6)
2. Cardiac conditions
    A. ETT – Required for all Ischemic heart disease. An abnormal ETT is defined as an inability to exceed 6 METS (beyond completion of Stage II or 6 minutes) on a standard Bruce protocol or the presence of Ischemic symptoms and/or signs (e.g. characteristic angina pain or a 1mm ST depression or elevation in 2 or more leads), inability to exceed 85% of age-predicted maximal heart rate, or ventricular dysrrythmia. Must be done biennially except for CABG

after 5 years, then must be done annually. (5-1:8)

B. ECG (EKG) – for all cardiac conditions. Minimum ejection fraction (or left ventricular ejection fraction) of 40% (50% for most valvular conditions). (5-1:6 through 5-1:27)

C. Alcohol Abuse – CAGE questionnaire. (9-1:28)

D. Anticoagulation therapy – INR (aka prothrombin time), must be done monthly, and maintain 2 to 3 and be stable (optimum normal values at 0.8 to 1.2).

E. Respiratory conditions

    i. OSA (Sleep Apnea) (5-2:18 through 5-2:22)

        a. Sleep study – Used to diagnose and comply with annual testing requirements.

            i. Epworth (5-2:19 and 5-2:20)

            ii. Sleep latency test

            iii. Wakefullness test

            iv. CPAP compliance report – required annually, must be at least 70%.

    ii. Any respiratory condition that will lead to decreased oxygen intake (examples include COPD, emphysema, interstitial lung diseases, chronic infectious diseases such as TB etc.) (5-2:4 through 5-2:6)

        a. Pulmonary Function Test - FEV1 minimum 65%, FVC minimum 60%, FEV1/FVC ratio minimum 65%.

        b. Pulse Oximetry – Minimum 92%

        c. ABG's – Minimum 65%.

    iii. Mental disorders – Folsteins test or MMSE (Mini-Mental State Exam). A score of 25 or greater out of 30 indicates they meet needed congnitive requirements.

    iv. Hearing (1-1:6, 2-1:4, 3-1:3, 3-1:4)

        a. Whisper test – perceives whispered voice at 5 feet in at least 1 ear.

        b. Audiometric test – Must have at least less than or equal to 40 db or better of the average at 500 Hz, 1000 Hz and 2000 hz. in ANSI values.

        c. To convert from ISO to ANSI, subtract, 14 from the hearing loss at 500 Hz, 10 from the hearing loss at 1000 Hz, and 8.5 from the hearing loss at 2000 Hz. Then add those numbers up, and divide by 3 to obtain the avg. hearing loss in ANSI (note that there are no negative numbers used in this determination. Anything that is negative, would be added in as a 0).

    v. UA – Required on all exams! (3-1:9 through 3-1:14)

        a. Specific Gravity – Normal 1.005 to 1.030 (optimum is 1.020).

        b. Protein – Negative

c. Blood – Negative

d. Glucose – Negative

Counseling Requirements

1. General counseling is required for non-compliance with treatment, side effects and interactions of medications, fatigue while driving etc.

2. Diabetes – for those with an exemption, council the driver to carry a form of rapidly absorbing glucose, self-monitoring kit, and to follow the requirement of the exemption including self-monitoring blood glucose levels 1 hour before driving and 1 time every 4 hours. The driver should also plan to submit blood glucose monitoring logs at the time of the examination to the medical examiner. (7-1:6)

3. Vision – Those who need corrective lenses, bring a spare pair of glasses. Contact users should also have a spare pair of glasses. Driver's who use monovision (one contact lens for distance, and one for near vision) cannot certify and must be counseled that this is not allowed by the FMCSA. (3-1:3)

4. Hearing aides – should bring a spare power source (3-1:4)

5. 12-hour rule – Many OTC decongestants and narcotic cough syrups cause drowsiness. A driver should not drive for 12 hours following using such medication. (5-2:7, 5-2:14)

6. History of DVT – Inform driver of risks of prolonged inactivity.

Waivers, Exemptions and SPE

1. Diabetic Waiver (49 CFR 391.64) – grandfathered program that has been discontinued but there still exists a small number of waivers, which were granted within the driver population. (2-1:6)

2. Diabetic Exemption – If the driver is an insulin dependant diabetic, they may apply for an exemption from the FMCSA, exemption program. To apply, the driver will need contact information to obtain information on the exemption program, a copy of the "Medical Certification Card" and "Medical Examination (Long) Form" both marked "accompanied by a insulin waiver/exemption". It will take up to 6 months for the process ot be completed (they may also apply for a State exemption which can be obtained much quicker, but they would then only be able to drive intrastate until the Federal exemption is granted). Once granted, they will have to present this to the examiner, including all stipulations identified within the exemption (testing 1 hour before driving, and every 4 hours, maintaining logs, having a rapidly absorbable form of glucose with them while driving). The exemption is good for 2 years (although they may only be certified for 1 year). (2-1:6, appendix)

3. Vision exemption – If the driver does not meet the minimum vision requirements to drive a CMV (see Non discretionary standard/ Vision above), they may apply for a vision exemption in the same manner listed above for "diabetic exemption". Again, they must be provided a copy of both their "Medical Certification Card" and Medical Examination (Long) Form" marked "accompanied by a vision waiver/ exemption". (3-1:3, appendix)

4. Neurologic waiver – for minor MS and Malignant tumors (marked on the medical certification card and examination form "accompanied by a neurologic waiver/

exemption). (7-1:14, appendix)

5. SPE (49 CFR 391.49) – Required for loss of limb or limb impairment (with a fixed deficit). The first, second and third digits are most important for prehensal ability and grip strength, with the fourth and fifth being less important. When the driver is missing only a part of their hand, it is a best practice decision for the CME to determine if the drivers grib strength and prehensal ability is adequate enough to drive a CME. Such conditions as CTS with a week hand grip do not require an SPE (not a fixed deficit).

    A. If the driver is found to need an SPE, the CME must mark this on the "Medical Certification Card" and "Medical Examination Form" (Long Form) "accompanied by an SPE". Copies of the card and exam form must be given to the driver so that hey may apply for the SPE at one of the 4 regional centers. The driver may apply at the local DMV but if granted, they are only able to drive intrastate.

    B. The SPE is good for 2 years. The driver may be certified for 2 years as long as there are no other conditions or treatments that would effect this. (7-1:6 and 7-1:7)

Disqualifying Conditions (Temporary and Permanent)

The examiner must always take into account the condition itself and its severity and symptoms, the progression and episodic nature, and its treatment (side effects and limitations).

1. Diabetes – Insulin dependent without an exemption or waiver. (1-1:5, 2-1:5 and 2-1:6)
2. Epilepsy – Always (see section on waiting periods/seizure disorders above for further understanding). (1-1:5, 2-1:9, 2-1:14, 7-1:11)
3. Mental disorders
    A. Schizophrenia – Always (2-1:14)
    B. Flat or blunt effect – Always
    C. Active psychosis – Always (2-1:14 and 2-1:15)
    D. Multiple personalities – DQ probable but no guidance exists. (2-1:12)
4. Active drug or alcohol abuse – Always (1-1:6, , 7-1:9, 7-1:11, 9-1:2, 9-1:9, 9-1:14,9-1:16, 9-1:18, 9-1:19, , 9-1:21, 9-1:28)
5. Vision
    A. Monocular driver – Always without a waiver or exemption. (3-1:2)
    B. Any driver that does not meet minimum vision requirement as defined above in section entitled "Non discretionary standard/Vision", who does not have a waiver or exemption.
6. Blood Pressure – Stage 3 until it is below 140/90. Also, if the driver is provided with a 1 time 3-month certificate, and the 3 months expires prior to them lowering their blood pressure below 140/90. At this point, the driver should undergo a new exam also. (3-1:5 through 3-1:8)
7. Pulse Rates – When above 100 or below 60 (truly a best practice decision) (3-1:8)
8. Cardiac/Vascular Conditions – Most are best practice decision. See sections on waiting periods, required medical testing, and required medical clearance. Any

chronic (developmental, acquired) symptomatic condition may be disqualifying.

    A. ICD – Always disqualifying. (5-1:12)

    B. Grade 3 or above murmur. (5-1:3)

    C. Left ventricular hypertrophy if does not meet minimum required testing requirements, or is symptomatic. (3-1:7)

    D. Cor pulmonale – same as left ventricular hypertrophy (5-2:17)

    E. Any condition that does not meet minimum testing requirements (See section on required testing)

    F. AAA or thoracic aneurysm that exceeds 5 cm (3.5 cm for thoracic aneurysm) or there is a greater than .5 cm increase in size over a 6 month time frame (5-1:28)

    G. Intermittent claudication – DQ if pain at rest. (5-1:28)

9. Respiratory conditions

    A. TB during active treatment (5-1:9)

    B. Chronic TB treated with Streptomycin (5-1:9)

    C. COPD with cough syncope (5-2:13)

    D. 2 or more spontaneous pneumothorax on the same side. (5-2:13)

    E. Bronchiectasis with hemoptysis. (5-1:8)

    F. Narcolepsy (5-2:23)

    G. All other conditions that do not meet testing requirements.

10. Abdominal, GU and other medical conditons. (6-1:1 through 6-:6)

    A. Renal Failure

    B. End stage kidney disease

    C. Hernias – non reducible and symptomatic (pain on exertion).

    D. Hematologic, GI, GU disorders based on severity, episodic nature and side effects of treatment.

    E. Neoplastic disease – Usually DQ during active treatment.

11. Orthopedic

    A. Loss or impairment of limb (fixed deficit), without SPE. (7-1:6)

    B. Any current limitation or disability that may impact the safe operation of a CMV (Best Practices).

    C. There are no defined range of motion requirements for any joint in the human body. It is a "Best Practice" decision by the CME as to whether or not the driver is able to safely operate a CMV with any limitations that may exist.

12. Neurologic (7-1:7 through 7-1:15)

    A. Legally incompetent

    B. Major psychiatric disorder

    C. Aphasia, Alexia,

D. Dementia – All
E. Cranial Neuralgia
F. Diplopia, and Oscillopsia
G. Nonfunctioning Labrinth
H. Amnesia
I. Chronic cluster HA
J. Migraines with neurologic deficits
K. Miniere's disease
L. Hemineglect
M. Heminopia
N. Many Neuromuscular diseases (understand peripherial neuropathy is disqualifying except if it only exhibits a hot/cold deficit)
O. Brain tumors
P. Parkinson's disease
Q. Seizures – discussed
R. Cerebellar degeneration with Ataxia
S. Cerebellar ataxia
T. Idiopathic CNS hypersomnolence and Primary Alveolar Hyperventilation syndrome
U. RLS – DOES
V. Severe TBI
W. TIA on anticoagulation therapy
X. Any other neurologic condition that has not fully recovered, is not well controlled or has not met minimum waiting periods

13. Active case of drug or alcohol addiction – Always. (9-1:27 through 9-1:29).

Allowable Hours Of Service For Drivers

Drivers must follow three maximum duty limits at all times;

1. 14 hour driving window limit
2. 11 hour driving limit
3. 60 hour/7 day and 70 hour/8 day duty limits

   8 hour limit since off-duty or sleeper period of at least 30 minutes (mostly applied to cross-country and regional drivers)

   There is a provision for a 34 hour "Restart" under certain conditions

   Work that is not driving is considered and must be included (such as working a second job)

Definitions For Hours Of Service

14- Hour Driving/Duty Window:

Considered a daily limit but not based on 24 hour period. Allowed a period of 14 consecutive hours in which to drive up to 11 hours after being off duty for 10 or more consecutive hours. 14 hour period begins at the start of any work. Once you reach 14 hours, you can not drive again until you have been off for 10 consecutive hours.

11-Hour Driving Limit:

During the 14 consecutive hour work period, you are only allowed to drive for a total of 11 hours. Note that to drive past 8 hours at any one time you must have at least 30 minutes off-duty.

60-Hour/7 Day & 70-Hour/8 Day Limit:

In addition to the other limits already explained, is the 60/70-hour limits based on a 7 or 8 day period.

Considered the "weekly" limit. The limits is based on a **"floating"** 7 or 8 day period. The oldest day's hours drops off at the end of the day when you calculate the total **on-duty time** for the past 7 or 8 days.

Driver's must comply with the previous driving limits and follow one of these two periods for driving.

Work that is not driving must be included (such as loading or unloading, inspection, maintaining logs etc. Also includes a second job such as working as a bartender, or in construction for example, during off hours).

Once they have reached a duty limit, the driver may not drive!

<u>**Disqualifying Medications and Medications of Concern**</u>

1. **Methadone** (Symoron, dolophine, Amidone, Methadose, Physeptone, Heptadon) - is always disqualifying. (1-1:6, 2-1:3, 9-1:10, appendix)

   Other medications used in the treatment of alcohol or drug abuse such as **Antabuse,** Saboxone, Naltrexone, if used for the treatment of alcohol or drug abuse are always disqualifying (these medications are occasionally used for the treatment of other conditions such as headaches, and if so the CME may choose to qualify the driver with medical clearance…Best Practice decision). (1-1:6, appendix)

2. **Chantix** – used for smoking cessation, is always disqualifying (see section on waiting periods for further understanding). (appendix)

3. All anti seizure medications when used to treat seizures will disqualify the driver (many are used for the treatment of other conditions and if the condition does not disqualify the driver, you may choose to certify the driver if they have medical clearance…Best Practice decision) (appendix)

   The medications include Diamox (acetaxolamide), Tegretol (Atretol, Epitol, Tegretol XR, Carbatrol, or Acetazolamide), Klonopin (Clonazepam), Valium (Diazepam), Zarontin (Ethosurzimide), Neurontin (Gabapentin), Limictal (Lamotrigine), Phenobarbital (Luminal, Solfoton, Mebaral), Dilantin (Cerebyx, Phenytoin sodium), Mysoline (Primidone), Depakene (Depakote, Valproic acid), Topamax (Topiramate).

4. Insulin dependent diabetics without a waiver or exemption cannot be qualified (refer to section on waivers and exemptions for further understanding). Insulin preparations come under a variety of names including Humalin, Novalog, Apidra, Belosulin, and others. They are typically injectable preparations except for **Exubra**, which is an inhaled insulin. Most non insulin medications (remember

you may certify the driver and it does not require a waiver or exemption) are oral medications except for **Byetta** (an injectable non insulin), and they include Metformin (Glucophage), Precose, Glucovance, Avandia, Glucotrol, Diabeta, Dymelor, and others. (appendix)

5. Mental or Psychiatric Medications (2-1:15, appendix)
   A. Benzodiazepines – Used to treat anxiety, but also used for numerous other purposes, such as an anti seizure medications, as muscle relaxants etc. The only Benzo that may be used for the treatment of a mental or psychiatric disorder (anxiety) is **Buspirone** (Ansial, Aniced, Anxiron, Axoren, Bespar, **Buspar**, Buspimen, Buspinol, Buspisal, Narol, Spamilan, Spitomin, Sorbon).
      i. If the Benzo is used for the treatment of another condition that is not in itself disqualifying, you may choose to certify with medical clearance (Best Practice decision).
      ii. Examples of disqualifying Benzodiazepines (when used for the treatment of anxiety) include Xanax (Alpraxolam), Lexotan (Bromazepam), Librium (Chlordiazepoxide), Klonopin (Clonazepam), Balium (Diazepam), ProSom (Extazolam), Ativan (Lorazepam), Serax (Oxazepam), Halcion (Triazolam).
   B. Anti-depressants – Only 2nd generation will qualify with medical clearance. The FMCSA considers SSRI's and SNRI's as second generation only. Tricyclic's and MAOI's as well as all the atypical anti depressants are considered 1st generation.
      i. SSRI's (Selective Serotonin Reuptake Inhibitors) – Include **Celexa** (Citalopram), Lexapro (Escitalopram oxalate), **Paxil** (Proxetine), **Prozac** (Fluoxitine), **Zoloft** (Sertraline).
      ii. SNRI's (Selective Norepinephrine Reuptake Inhibitors) – Include Cymbalta (Duloxetine), **Effexor** (Venlafaxine), Pristiq (Desvenlafaxine).
      iii. MAOI's (Monoamine Oxidase Inhibitor) – Nardil (Phenelzine), Parnate (Tranylcypromine)
      iv. Tricyclics – Adapin (Doxepin), Anafranil (Clominpramine), **Elavil** (**Amitriptyline**, Typtozol), Norpramin (Desipramine), Pertofane, Desiparmine (Despramine), **Tofranil** (Imipramine), Vivactil (Protriptline).
      v. Special considerations – Driver's taking **Wellbutrin (Buproprion),** a unicyclic anti depressant, may be qualified, Also, if the driver is taking **amitriptyline**, 25mg (lowest dose) only at night, they may be qualified. If the driver is taking Lithium (a Benzo that is commonly prescribed for Bi polor disorder), they may be qualified after a 3 month waiting period.
   C. Hypnotics – Only short acting compounds with a half-life of 5 hours (lowest dose) and only for a maximum of 2 weeks. Examples of Hypnotics include Welldorm (Chloral betaine), Nytol (Medinex), Sominex (Phenegran), Sonata (Zaleplon) and Ambien (Stilnoct, Zolpidem).

D. Neuroleptics (anti psychotics) – Extreme caution required for certification. May indicate active psychosis (disqualifying condition) and there are notable side effects. They may be used in the treatment of other conditions and if there is no psychosis, they may be considered for certification. Examples of neuroleptics include Abilify, Droperidol, Prolizin, Haldol, **Seroquel**, Zeprexa, Symbyaz, (combination of Prozac and Zyprexa).

E. Stimulants – May only be used for the treatment of ADHD and ADD. Include Focalin (Dexmethzlphenidate HCL), Dexedrine (Dextrostat), Concerta (Methylphenidate), Ritalin, Adderall. If used for another reason these medications would disqualify the driver.

F. Any medication used to treat a disqualifying condition would of course disqualify a driver. An example is **Sinimet** which is used to treat Parkinson's disease.

6. Pharmacology Other

A. Narcotic medications (most are opiods and synthetic opoid derivatives, and all are scheduled drugs) must have clearance from treating providers. Concern would also be for the condition that they are prescribed for. Examples include Oxycodone, Oxycotin, Hydrocodone, and others which are used to treat chronic pain. If the driver does not exhibit any side effects that would interfere with the safe operation of a CMV, you may certify the driver with medical clearance as long as your exam findings or the condition itself do not disqualify them.

B. **Bentyl** is used for the treatment of IBS. As long as there are no side effects and the condition is well managed, then the driver may be certified.

C. Anticoagulants – Used to treat numerous cardiovascular problems. Remember waiting periods and always consider what they are treating in making a decision. Examples of anticoagulants include **Cumadin**, **Warfin**, Prodaxa (does not require monthly INR testing). Low dose ASA is not considered an anti-coagulate.

D. **Methotrexate** is used in the treatment of cancer, autoimmune disease (such as RA). Predisposes to infection, nausea, abdominal pain, fatigue, fever, dizziness, acute pheumonitis and rarely pulmonary fibrosis

NOTE: ALL NON-REGULATED CONDITIONS AND MEDICATIONS IN BOLD PRINT HAVE BEEN SPECIFICALLY MENTIONED IN THE ON-LINE HANDBOOK AND/OR THE SAMPLE TRAINING PROGRAM (OFTEN IN SAMPLE QUESTIONS AND PRACTICE SCENARIOS). IT IS RECOMMENDED THAT YOU PAY SPECIAL ATTENTION TO THESE AS THEY ARE MORE LIKELY TO BE TESTED.

NOTES

NRCME PRACTICE TEST

Please choose the "most correct" answer for the following questions. You must make your decision only from the information provided. Only one (1) answer may be chosen for each question.

1. The driver was recently prescribed insulin for the control of his diabetes. The examiner would?
   a. Certify the driver for 2 years with medical clearance provided by their treating physician.
   b. Certify the driver for 1 year with medical clearance provided by their treating physician.
   c. Permanently disqualify the driver.
   d. The driver is disqualified until the driver obtains a diabetic exemption.

2. The driver first perceives a whispered voice at 5 feet in his right ear and 4 feet in his left ear. All other aspects of his physical examination are unremarkable. The examiner would?
   a. Permanently disqualify the driver because he "failed" the whispered voice" test.
   b. Certify the driver for 2 years.
   c. Certify the driver for 1 year.
   d. Require an audiometric test to determine the extent of hearing loss in his left ear.

3. The medical examiner notices that the driver has recently been prescribed "Chantix" to help him stop smoking while reviewing the drivers history. The driver is?
   a. Qualified for 2 years if the rest of his exam is within normal limits.
   b. Provided a 1-time 3 month certificate so that the examiner can monitor how well the driver is doing with smoking cessation.
   c. Disqualified until it has been confirmed he is no longer taking Chantix and that he has suffered no ill effects from withdrawal from the medication.
   d. Qualified for only 1 year while taking Chantix, and then he may be qualified for 2 years once he no longer needs the medication.

4. The driver reports for an examination 6 weeks after suffering a mild heart attack and presents a note from the cardiologist stating that he is able to return to work immediately without restriction. Included within the note, the cardiologist provides recent testing information showing that the driver had an ETT that showed that the driver was able to reach 12 METS during the test. His ECG showed an ejection fraction of 65%. The examination of the driver was unremarkable. The examiner should?
   a. Temporarily disqualify the driver.
   b. Qualify the driver for 1 year.
   c. Qualify the driver for 2 years.
   d. Consult with the cardiologist to determine if the driver suffers from angina.

5. A driver provides an audiometric test listing the following findings:

500 Hz: 35 Right ear; 40 Left ear
1000 Hz: 40 Right ear; 45 Left ear
2000 Hz: 40 Right ear; 45 Left ear
4000Hz: 50 Right ear; 50 Left ear

The medical examiner should:
   a. Disqualify the driver because he does not meet minimum hearing requirements to drive.
   b. Certify the driver for 2 years.
   c. Certify the driver for 1 year.
   d. Require the driver to obtain a hearing exemption.

6. The medical examiner notes that the driver is taking Metformin for the treament of diabetes, Antabuse, and Crestor to reduce serum cholesterol levels. He reports no side effects from any of the medications. The rest of the examination is unremarkable. The examiner should:
   a. Disqualify the driver.
   b. Request clearance for all medications due to side effects.
   c. Certify the driver for 1 year.
   d. Certify the driver for 2 years.

7. The following are symptoms of Congestive Heart Failure EXCEPT:
   a. Shortness of breath on exertion or at rest in severe cases.
   b. Need to urinate at night
   c. Headache
   d. Swelling in the ankles and the abdomen.

8. During the examination, the examiner notices that the driver's peripheral vision is 70 degrees to the left and 80 degrees to the right. The examiner should?
   a. Qualify the driver for 2 years.
   b. Require the driver to obtain a vision exemption because of the limitation in the drivers left peripheral field.
   c. Disqualify the driver
   d. Have the driver consult with an Ophthalmologist to determine if the driver's peripheral vision, meet minimum standards.

9. During an examination, the examiner notices that the driver is distant, lacks eye contact and shows absolutely no emotional response during the exam. The examiners best response should be.
   a. Provide the driver with a "CAGE" questionnaire to determine if they suffer from alcoholism.
   b. Disqualify the driver and refer them to a mental health professional prior to consideration for certification.
   c. Certify the driver with a 1-time 3 month certificate to determine if there is any effect on the driver's ability to drive a CMV
   d. Require a skill performance evaluation to ascertain if the driver has any limitations with driving.

10. The driver reports that he had surgery to his cervical spine 2 years ago. It involved a fusion of C4, 5 and 6. He has recovered fully and been provided a release to return to work without restriction. He reports no pain and does not require medication of any kind. During the examination, the examiner notices that the driver exhibits only 30 degrees of cervical rotation to both the right and the left. The examiners best decision would be to:
    a. Certify the driver if trunk and neck rotation is determined to be sufficient to see his mirrors and change lanes while driving.
    b. Instruct the driver to apply for an SPE
    c. Instruct the driver to apply for an orthopedic exemption.
    d. Review the driving record of the driver to determine if he is safe to drive a CMV.

11. The driver admits to the use of marijuana for the treatment of his glaucoma, which is legal in the State he lives in. He provides medical documentation for the glaucoma indicating he is able to drive a truck. He began using the marijuana about three months ago. His current medical card has no limitations listed and is for 2 years. His certification examination is WNL. The medical examiner should?
    a. Disqualify the driver.
    b. Perform a urine drug collection and provide the release from the treating provider.
    c. Certify the driver for 1 year.
    d. Certify the driver for 2 years.

12. The driver has a blood pressure of 136/92. This is:
    a. Within normal limits and would not effect the drivers certification.
    b. Stage 1 Htn.
    c. Stage 2 Htn.
    d. Stage 3 Htn.

13. The driver reports for a new certification at a local trucking school. He reports in his history that he was treated for epilepsy 14 years ago but stopped taking medication on his own since his move to your area 11 years ago. He has not seen a neurologist in greater than 10 years and reports no seizures since then. The examiner should?
    a. Request medical clearance and if obtained the driver may be certified for 1 year.
    b. Request medical clearance and if obtained the driver may be certified for 2 years.
    c. Have the driver obain a neurologic waiver.
    d. Disqualify the driver.

14. A driver reports having been diagnosed with sleep apnea 3 years earlier. He reports seeing his "sleep doc" a few months ago and that he had a new sleep study. His exam is essentially normal other than he is overweight (BMI of 38.33). The best decision for the examiner is to:
    a. Disqualify the driver because he has sleep apnea.
    b. Certify the driver for 1 year.
    c. Certify the driver for 2 years.
    d. Provide a temporary certificate so that the driver may obtain required testing results and a CPAP compliance report.

15. A driver must exhibit a minimum of what % compliance of CPAP usage?
    a. 60%
    b. 70%
    c. 80%
    d. 100%

16. A driver is taking "Celexa" for the treatment by his PCP of what he calls a mild depression".
    He reports he has not considered or attempted suicide. The examiner should?
    a. Temporarily disqualify the driver until he obtains written clearance for the depression and the medication.
    b. Certify the driver for a period of 1 year.
    c. Certify the driver for a period of 2 years.
    d. Disqualify the driver until he is no longer requiring medication for the treatment of depression.

17. The driver reports for a re-certification examination. In his history he reports he was hospitalized 8 months ago for what was diagnosed as a "TIA". In addition he is being treated for and he has been taking coumadin to manage atrial fibrillation for which he has been treated for during the past two years. He provides a note from his cardiologist stating he has no restrictions and he may drive a CMV. The examiner would?
    a. Certify the driver for 1 year.
    b. Certify the driver for 2 years.
    c. Request an electrocardiogram.
    d. Disqualify the driver.

18. The driver marks "Injury and Illness in the past 5 years" in the history. He reports that he had a hunting accident where he suffered a left orbital fracture. He presents a note at the time of the examination from an ophthalmologist stating "may drive". His exam is unremarkable except for a limitation in peripheral vision in his left eye, which was inconclusive. His distance vision was 20/20 right and 20/40 left. The medical examiner should?
    a. Council the driver on the need for a vision exemption.
    b. Disqualify the driver pending vision exam to determine if it meets peripheral vision requirements
    c. Certify the driver for 1 year.
    d. Certify the driver for 2 years.

19. What minimum PaO2 level is necessary if the driver has an ABG due to a chronic respiratory disorder.
    a. 55%
    b. 60%
    c. 65%
    d. 70%

20. The driver is taking "Topomax" for the treatment of migraine headaches. He reports good management for his headaches and they never seem to interfere with his driving ability with the medication. The medical examiner should?
    a. Obtain medical clearance for the condition and the medication
    b. Disqualify the driver because he is taking an anti seizure medication.
    c. Certify the driver for 1 year.
    d. Certify the driver for 2 years.

21. The certification period for a driver who has a vision exemption is how long, and how long is the exemption good for.
    a. Certify for 1 year and the exemption must be renewed annually.
    b. Certify for 2 years and the exemption must be renewed annually.
    c. Certify for 1 year and the exemption must be renewed every 2 years.
    d. Certify for 2 years and the exemption must be renewed every 2 years.

22. What is the waiting period for "Viral encephalitis with early seizures"?
    a. 1 year
    b. 2 years
    c. 5 years
    d. 10 years

23. Can a driver be certified while taking "methadone" for chronic pain management?
    a. Yes with medical clearance for 1 year.
    b. Yes with medical clearance for 2 years.
    c. No, because use of methadone is always prohibited.
    d. No, because drivers are disqualified during chronic pain management.

24. A driver has a blood pressure of 168/112 confirmed during the examination. The driver would be?
    a. Disqualified
    b. Certified for 6 months
    c. Certified for 1 year
    d. Certified for 2 years.

25. How long would the driver be certified for if they are taking Micardis HCT for hypertension, who has a confirmed blood pressure of 148/96 at the time of the examination.
    a. 3 months
    b. 6 months
    c. 1 year
    d. 2 years

26. A driver with a history of diabetes, who is taking metforman, provides a note from his PCP that lists his A1c level as 10. His exam is essentially WNL including laboratory analysis except he is notably overweight. The medical examiner should?
    a. Disqualify the driver until his A1c level is less than 7.
    b. Disqualify the driver because he is an insulin dependant diabetic.
    c. Certify the driver for 1 year.
    d. Certify the driver for 2 years.

27. During the examination the driver has a positive "Babinski" reflex. The examiner should?
    a. Certify the driver for 1 year.
    b. Certify the driver for 2 years.
    c. Council the driver to obtain an SPE.
    d. Disqualify the driver until they have a neurological consult.

28. The driver marks yes for a history of "Lung disease, emphysema, asthma, chronic bronchitis", and lists that he uses an albuteral inhaler multiple times per week to control his asthma, and that it is worse in the spring and fall. Upon further questioning, he denies ever being hospitalized for his asthma and that he sees his PCP annually for a physical. The examiner should?
    a. Temporarily disqualify the driver until they obtain clearance from the PCP.
    b. Council the driver to obtain a respiratory waiver from the FMCSA.
    c. Certify the driver for 1 year.
    d. Certify the driver for 2 years.

29. All of the following are required components of all DOT medical examinations EXCEPT?
    a. Vision
    b. Hearing
    c. Blood Pressure
    d. Ophthalmoscopic examination

30. The driver lists they are using "Byetta" for control of their diabetes, along with dietary control. The rest of the examination is normal. The examiner should?
    a. Disqualify the driver because byetta is an insulin and they would need to obtain a diabetic exemption in order to drive a CMV.
    b. Provide a 1-time, 3-month certificate in order to obtain the drivers A1c level from their treating provider.
    c. Certify the driver for 1 year.
    d. Certify the driver for 2 years.

31. In order for the driver to obtain a vision exemption, the medical examiner must?
    a. Provide the driver only the medical certification card marked "temporarily disqualified", with a second box marked "reconsidered with a vision exemption".
    b. Provide the driver only the medical certification card marked "certified for 2 years, and also marked "accompanied by a vision waiver/exemption.
    c. Provide the driver the medical certification card and the long form both marked "certified for 2 years" and also marked "accompanied by a vision waiver/exemption.
    d. Provide the driver the medical certification card and long form both marked "certified for 1 year" and also marked "accompanied by a vision waiver/exemption.

32. The driver is on dialysis, and the examiner is unable to obtain a UA during the certification examination. The examiner should?
    a. Disqualify the driver
    b. Contact the treating provider to obtain clearance.
    c. Certify the driver for 1 year.
    d. Certify the driver for 2 years.

33. The driver reports for a re-certification examination 8 weeks after a having a triple by pass. He present a note from his treating provider stating that the driver is able to return to driving without restriction. Additionally, it mentions that the drivers results for his ETT were normal and his ECG showed a left ventricular ejection fraction of 75. The examiner should?
   a. Temporarily disqualify the driver until he has completed the required waiting period.
   b. Permanently disqualify the driver because his ejection fraction is too low.
   c. Certify the driver for 1 year only.
   d. Certify the driver for 2 years because he has medical clearance.

34. All of the following eye conditions may require the medical examiner to seek specialist evaluation except?
   a. Monovision
   b. Glaucoma
   c. Cataracts
   d. Macular Degeneration

35. The driver lists that he is taking "ambien" 10 mg as a sleep aide at night before bed, and has been taking this for 2 months. The medical examiner should
   a. Certify the driver for 1 year
   b. Certify the driver for 2 years.
   c. Obtain clearance from the treating provider prior to certification. If cleared to drive, the driver may be certified for 1 year.
   d. Temporarily disqualify the driver because he is taking a sedative hypnotic medication at a higher dose and for greater than 2 weeks.

36. A blood pressure of 166/92 would be?
   a. Considered normal
   b. Stage 1 hypertension
   c. Stage 2 hypertension
   d. Stage 3 hypertension

37. The driver is taking "Sinimet" for the treatment of Parkinson's disease. The medical examiner should?
   a. Disqualify the driver.
   b. Obtain medical clearance from a neurologist.
   c. Counsel the driver to obtain a neurological waiver
   d. Certify the driver for 1 year.

38. The driver uses hearing aides during the whisper test. He is able to hear at 5 feet on the right and 4 feet on the left.
   a. Send the driver for an audiometric test.
   b. Disqualify the driver.
   c. Certify the driver for 1 year.
   d. Certify the driver for 2 years.

39. The minimum acceptable spirometry values required to certify a driver are?
   a. FEV1 70%, FVC 65%, FEV1/FVC ratio 65%.
   b. FEV1 65%, FVC 60%, FEV1/FVC ratio 65%
   c. FEV1 65%, FVC 65%, FEV1/FVC ratio 65%
   d. FEV1 60%, FVC 60%, FEV1/FVC ratio 60%

40. A female driver presents for re-certification who is in her fourth day of menses with heavy bleeding. Her UA shows a Specific gravity of 1.020; Protein is +1; Blood is +4; Glucose is negative. All other aspects of her medical examination are within normal. The examiner should?
    a. Obtain medical clearance prior to certification
    b. Disqualify the driver
    c. Certify the driver for 1 year.
    d. Certify the driver for 2 years.

41. A driver presenting to your office marks down that he is taking "nitroglycerine" for angina and he has been doing so for a few years. Upon questioning he indicates that he has needed more recently because his episodes have become more frequent. Your best course of action is to?
    a. Council the driver to increase his dose of medication.
    b. Certify the driver for 1 year.
    c. Provide a 1-time, 3 month certificate to monitor his condition
    d. Disqualify the driver and refer him to his cardiologist for further evaluation.

42. Upon auscultation of the driver's abdomen, you hear a loud bruit. Palpation reveals a bounding pulsation below the sternal angle of the rib cage. You as an examiner may suspect?
    a. Hiatal hernia
    b. Renal artery stenosis
    c. Aortic Abdominal Aneurysm
    d. Gastrointestinal distress

43. The longest the medical examiner would certify a driver with a history of Stage 3 hypertension is?
    a. 3 months
    b. 6 months
    c. 12 months
    d. 24 months

44. The driver is taking "Wellbutrin", low dose, to help him stop smoking. He is provided a note from his PCP stating that he has no side effects and confirms that he is taking the medication for smoking cessation. The examiner would?
    a. Certify the driver for 2 years.
    b. Certify the driver for 1 year.
    c. Disqualify the driver because the medication is not allowed.
    d. Council the driver to only take the medication at night.

45. During the history the driver admits to taking "Benydril" for seasonal allergies. The examiner should?
    a. Council the driver to not take the medication for 12 hours prior to driving.
    b. Obtain medical clearance from the driver's PCP that he/she can drive.
    c. Disqualify the driver until he is no longer taking Benydril.
    d. Provide a 1-time, 3 month certificate to determine the medications effect on the driver.

46. The driver has a history of a moderate Traumatic Brain Injury that occurred 3 years ago as a result of a car accident. He reports he has fully recovered and provides a note from his neurologist stating that he suffered no seizures and that he is able to return to driving. He does not list any medications in his history. The examiner should?
    a. Disqualify the driver.
    b. Require the driver to take a "Folstein's mini mental state exam".
    c. Certify the driver for 1 year.
    d. Certify the driver for 2 years.

47. The driver marks that he has suffered a seizure that occurred 5 months earlier. Upon further questioning, he indicates it was a result of a medication reaction, he only had one event, and that he did not require any medication. Within a few days, the driver is able to confirm this information from the neurologist who examined him. The examiner should?
    a. Disqualify the driver because he has a history of epilepsy.
    b. Disqualify the driver because he has not completed the 6 months waiting period.
    c. Certify the driver for 2 years.
    d. Certify the driver for 1 year.

48. The driver reports a suicide attempt 10 months earlier following the break up of his marriage. He noted seeing a psychiatrist and he takes citalopram daily and he reports he feels fine now and is moving on with his life. He provides a release from his doctor that he may return to work without restrictions. The medical examiner's should?
    a. Disqualify the driver.
    b. Require a CAGE questionnaire.
    c. Certify the driver for 1 year.
    d. Certify the driver for 2 years.

49. The driver lists "Synthroid" for the treatment of hypothyroidism. He has been taking it for about 6 months and feel fine now. His examination is essentially normal. The examiners best course of action is to?
    a. Request medical clearance for the medication prior to certification.
    b. Certify the driver for 1 year.
    c. Certify the driver for 2 years.
    d. Council the drive that he needs to apply for an endocrine exemption.

50. A 48 year old male driver presents for a certification examination. He reports in his history a back injury that had occurred 4 years earlier. He states that he was out of work following back surgery for over a year, but since has returned to driving and his last certification was good for 2 years. He lists as his only medication Oxycodone, which he takes only as needed. He reports seeing his "pain doctor" every few months for evaluation. He also reports he has had a steroid injection (series of 3) about a year ago which "helped a lot". The examiner should?
    a. Request medical clearance.
    b. Certify the driver for 1 year.
    c. Certify the driver for 2 years.
    d. Disqualify the driver.

51. A driver reports for an examination with a history of using cumadin to treat Atrial Fibrillation. He presents with medical clearance from his cardiologist stating he may drive and his most recent INR is 2.5. The examiner would?
    a. Provide a 1 time 3-month certificate to obtain an A1c reading. If below 10, the driver may be certified for 1 year.
    b. Disqualify the driver because his INR is too high.
    c. Certify the driver for 1 year.
    d. Certify the driver for 2 years.

52. The driver's UA shows a specific gravity of 1.030, Protein is negative, Blood shows a trace amount, and Glucose is 2000. The most significant area of concern for the examiner would be if the driver suffers from?
    a. Kidney stones
    b. Bladder cancer
    c. A UTI
    d. Diabetes

53. The driver admits during the examination that he drinks frequently, usually only on the weekends, but he may "down 12 to 14" beers to help him unwind. The examiner provides a "CAGE" questionnaire and the driver scores a 1 on the questionnaire. The rest of the examination is unremarkable. The examiner should?
    a. Disqualify the driver until he has undergone evaluation by a Substance Abuse Professional.
    b. Certify the driver for 1 year if he agrees to attend AA meetings.
    c. Certify the driver for 1 year with a clearance from his PCP.
    d. Certify the driver for 2 years.

54. During a history the driver admits that he has been treated in the last year for tuberculosis, had a chest X-ray and took an antibiotic whose name he could not remember. He reports that he was ok and was cleared to drive. The examiner should:
    a. Certify the driver for 1 year.
    b. Certify the driver for 2 years.
    c. Disqualify the driver until he/she receives medical clearance and required testing.
    d. The driver is permanently disqualified because he has TB.

55. A driver reports with a medical report from his cardiologist providing clearance for the driver that had a successful catheter ablation 8 months earlier to treat his "Wolf Parkinson White syndrome" and his latest electrocardiogram is normal. Examination shows no significant abnormalities in rhythm and timing of the cardiac cycle and the rest of his examination is unremarkable. The examiner should:
    a. Certify the driver for 1 year.
    b. Certify the driver for 2 years.
    c. Temporarily disqualify the driver because they have not met the required waiting period for the condition.
    d. Permanently disqualify the driver.

56. The driver lists in his history that he has diabetes and is taking insulin. He provides his exemption that was granted last year consequent to his last certification exam, and a log indicating that he has monitored his sugar levels. The CME should:
    a. Disqualify the driver because he did not reapply for his exemption.
    b. Certify the driver for 1 year.
    c. Certify the driver for 2 years.
    d. Request medical clearance from the treating provider.

57. A driver exhibits the following finding when presenting for examination (see Illustration 1 below). The examiners next step as a result of this finding would be?
    a. The finding is normal, and the driver may be certified for 2 years if the rest of the examination is normal.
    b. Provide the driver with a 1 time 3-month certificate to see if the condition worsens.
    c. Obtain a specialists opinion regarding the condition.
    d. The condition will permanently disqualify the driver.

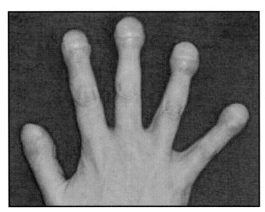

Illustration 1

58. The driver lists a history of hypertension and diabetes on his history. Upon further questioning he comments that his wife complains of his loud snoring. His current list of medications includes lisinopril, glucovance, and symvastatin. His examination shows a BP of 136/82. The rest of his examination is unremarkable other than his BMI is a 42.26. The examiner should:
    a. Certify the driver for 1 year.
    b. Certify the driver for 2 years.
    c. Request an clearance from his treating provider because of the hypertension and diabetes.
    d. Request that the driver have a "sleep study" because of his BMI and history of hypertension and diabetes and loud snoring.

59. The driver takes "Bentyl" for his Irritable Bowl Syndrome. He reports that the condition is well managed and he has had no difficulty driving over the past few years. The examiner should:
    a. Disqualify the drive because Bentyl is a disqualifying medication.
    b. Obtain clearance for the driver's condition from their treating provider.
    c. Certify the driver for 1 year.
    d. Certify the driver for 2 years.

60. A female driver reports for a re-certification examination. She is 36 years old and has a benign history. Upon examination she shows nothing abnormal other than her UA shows a significant amount of blood within her urine. Upon further testing she indicates that she is in the middle of her menstrual cycle. The examiner should:
    a. Certify the driver for 1 year
    b. Certify the driver for 2 years.
    c. Provide a temporary certificate and obtain clearance from the driver's gynecologist.
    d. Order a CBC to determine if the driver suffers from a UTI prior to certification.

61. The waiting period for a driver who has attempted suicide is?
    a. There is no waiting period.
    b. 3 months
    c. 6 months
    d. 12 months

62. A driver reports for examination 6 years post having a triple bi-pass surgery. He presents a release from his recent visit to the cardiologist that states that he has no restrictions from driving. A copy of his ETT that was done 2 years ago was provided, and the driver was able to reach 12 mets. His examination is unremarkable. The certified medical examiners best choice would be to:
    a. Certify the driver for 3 months to allow him to have another ETT to complete his annual required testing requirements.
    b. Certify the driver for 1 year.
    c. Certify the driver for 2 years.
    d. Disqualify the driver because his ETT did not meet minimum requirements.

63. A driver reports for a new certification at a local trucking school. He noted in his history that he is being treated for PTSD at the local VA hospital. He lists his medications as Symbyax (a combination medication of Prozac and Zyprexa), and trazadone, which is used as a sleep aide. In the treating physicians note, he provides clearance, and reports that the driver has not suffered a psychotic episode since being medicated and that the driver does not suffer any side effects that would interfere with driving from either medication. The examiner should:
    a. Certify the driver for 1 year.
    b. Certify the driver for 2 years.
    c. Disqualify the driver
    d. Provide the driver a CAGE questionnaire and if they score a 3 or above, they may be certified for 1 year.

64. The following symptoms are symptoms of core pulmonale except:
    a. Shortness of breath
    b. Ascites
    c. Pedal edema
    d. Night sweats

65. The driver reports of history of COPD. He also notes during his examination that he smokes a pack and a half of cigarettes daily. He has been treated by a pulmonologist for a few years now but he insists he is able to drive safely. He lists that he is taking Spiriva daily as well as his "water pill" which he cannot remember the name of, for high blood pressure. His examination reveals notable wheezing in all lung fields upon auscultation, a BMI of 34.23, and the rest of his examination is unremarkable. The examiner should:

    a. Request a Sleep Study.

    b. Request a Pulmonary Function Test

    c. Certify the driver for 1 year.

    d. Certify the driver for 2 years.

66. The picture of a driver is seen in Illustration 2 below. The driver exhibits symptoms of:

    a. Peripheral vascular disease

    b. Central cynosis

    c. Ascites

    d. A cranial nerve abnormality.

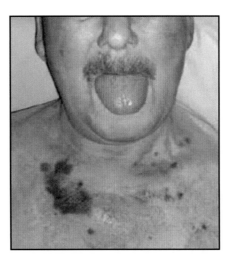

Illustration 2

67. During the vision portion of the examination, the driver reports significant difficulty in his peripheral vision, and is limited to 30 degrees on the left and 60 degrees on the right. Of the following diagnosis, which one could cause a restriction of peripheral vision?

    a. Macular degeneration

    b. Cataracts

    c. Glaucoma

    d. Diabetic retinopathy

68. The driver is taking Streptomycin for the treatment of chronic tuberculosis. His history reveals that he has not been symptomatic within the past year. He reports no significant fatigue and his examination findings are unremarkable. He provides a note from his treating physician that indicates that he may drive a truck. Office notes including his most recent X-ray, and pulmonary function tests are also provided for the examiners review. The X-ray shows a few discrete nodules, without any other abnormal findings. The PFT has an FEV1 of 75, FVC of 70 and an FEV/FVC ration of 75. The examiner should:
    a. Certify the driver for 1 year
    b. Certify the driver for 2 years
    c. Disqualify the driver
    d. Request additional information regarding any recent tuberculin skin testing performed on the driver to determine if it is active or inactive.

69. While completing the examination, the examiner notices that the driver has noticeable pain in his lower back during lumbar flexion. The driver then indicates that he has had a recent lower back injury and is under active treatment for a low back strain. He has been released to return to work but has current limitations of lifting anything greater than 10 lbs, with frequent bending, and with prolonged sitting. All other aspects of the examination are unremarkable. The examiner should.
    a. Certify the driver for 3 months and highlight the drivers current limitations to be followed by their employer.
    b. Temporarily disqualify the driver until they are released from active treatment and are able to perform all required functions of truck driving.
    c. Certify the driver for 1 year.
    d. Certify the driver for 2 years.

70. The driver is unable to raise his left arm above shoulder height during the examination but is adamant that he is able to drive a truck. His previous examiner has certified him for 2 years and he reports he has had no difficulty driving over the past two years and that he has suffered from this problem for many years. He also reports that he does not require treatment and has not seen a physician in many years. The rest of his examination is unremarkable. The examiner should.
    a. Certify the driver for 2 years
    b. Certify the driver for 1 year
    c. Request a copy of the drivers "driving record" from his current employer prior to making a determination.
    d. Require a orthopedic evaluation to determine if the driver requires a SPE.

71. Upon examination, the driver is a well developed athletic type female. Her examination reveals a BP of 98/62 and a pulse of 56. She reports she is a triathlete and she runs, swims and bikes daily. The examiners best decision regarding her certification would be:
    a. Temporarily disqualify the driver due to her pulse rate being below 60, and obtain medical clearance.
    b. Certify the driver for 3 months and reevaluate the drivers pulse rate at that time.
    c. Obtain a "CBC" and "Pulmonary Function Test" to determine if the driver's current level of apparent fitness corresponds with testing findings.
    d. Certify the driver for 2 years.

72. A driver is unable to identify most of the numbers that are within the ishihara's color blind test, but is able to identify the specific colors of "signal red", "signal green" and "signal yellow" for the examiner when he is shown the colors separately. The examiner should:
    a. Disqualify the driver because he is colorblind.
    b. Refer the driver to an Opthamologist for further evaluation.
    c. The driver must be certified for only 1 year because of they are colorblind.
    d. The examiner may certify the driver for 2 years if all other aspects of their examination are within normal limits.

73. A driver reports a history of being treated for alcoholism many years prior. He has attended AA meetings for years, and he reports not drinking for over 5 years. He also does not take any medication to control his alcoholism. His last certification performed a year ago was good for 1 year due to the fact he takes hypertensive medication. His examination is unremarkable. The examiner provides a CAGE questionnaire and the driver scores a 0 out of 4. The best certification decision would be to.
    a. Certify the driver for 1 year.
    b. Certify the driver for 2 years.
    c. Temporarily disqualify the driver until that have been to a SAP.
    d. Temporarily disqualify the driver until you receive clearance from their Primary Care Physician.

74. A 67 year-old male driver has a history of hypertension and diabetes listed on his examination form. He lists lisinopril, HCT, pravastatin, metformin and aricept that was written on the form by his wife, another driver who has attended the examination with her husband. She mentions that she and her husband work as team drivers and she is always with him. Upon further questioning, they seem evasive concerning the reasoning for the use of aricept. The driver's wife also seems to try and answer many of the questions asked by the examiner during the exam. The rest of the exam is unremarkable. The examiners best decision would be to:
    a. Certify the driver for 2 years.
    b. Certify the driver for 1 year.
    c. Temporarily disqualify the driver to obtain medical information for the use of Aricept.
    d. Refer the driver to an SAP because he currently suffers from an active case of alcoholism.

75. A driver who undergoes angioplasty has a waiting period of how long?
    a. 1 week
    b. 1 month
    c. 2 months
    d. 3 months

76. The urine analysis that is performed during the DOT physical examination is primarily to assess?
    a. Heart and Kidney function
    b. Kidney and Bladder disease
    c. Drug Use
    d. Kidney function and diabetes

77. All of the following meet the FMCSA definition of epilepsy except:
    a. 2 or greater unexplained episodes
    b. 2 or more explained episodes (such as from a high fever or a medication reaction).
    c. Use of anti-seizure medication to control seizures
    d. A clinical diagnosis of epilepsy from a neurologist.

78. A driver who has a PCI procedure 2 weeks ago, has medical clearance from a cardiologist, and an ETT that is at 12 Mets, and ECG with a EF of 55%, may be certified for how long?
    a. 3 to 6 months
    b. 1 year
    c. 2 years
    d. They may not be certified because they have not met their minimum waiting period.

79. A 28-year old African American driver reports for examination. His list of medications includes ibuprofen OTC used prn for aches and pains, and Folic Acid. He provides a note from his Hemotologist that provides a release to drive without restriction, that he has a diagnosis of sidkle-cell anemia, which in the note he reports has been well managed and stable without crisis for a number of years. His latest CBC does not demonstrate any significant anemia. The driver is alert and coherent and the rest of the exam is WNL. The examiners best decision would be to:
    a. Disqualify the driver
    b. Have the driver complete a Folsteins mini mental health questionnaire to determine his cognitive ability.
    c. Certify the driver for 2 years
    d. Certify the driver for 1 year

80. The driver reports for examination 3 ½ months after being provided a 3-month certificate for having Stage 1 hypertension. His list of medications has not changed and he is taking lisinopril, and crestor for high blood pressure. He reports not seeing his PCP or done anything else since his last exam. A new exam is performed, and his blood pressure is 148/88 confirmed with a second reading. The examiner should:
    a. Provide the driver with another 3-month certificate to lower his blood pressure and instruct him to see his PCP.
    b. Provide the driver with the remainder of his 1-year certificate dated from the original examination.
    c. Provide the driver with a 1-year certificate from the date of the current examination.
    d. Disqualify the driver.

81. A 43-year old male driver reports for a re-certification examination. His previous certification was good for 2 years. His history is benign. Further questioning reveals an appendectomy 8 years ago, and no current medications. His examination is as follows:
   - Vision is 20/30 left; 20/20 right; 20/20 both; not color blind; peripherial vision is 80 left, 80 right.
   - Whisper test is 5 right; 4 left
   - BP 148/88; pulse: 86
   - UA: Specific Gravity: 1.010; Protein: trace; Blood: Negative; Sugar: Negative.
   - The rest of the examination is unremarkable.

   The examiners best decision would be to:
   - a. Disqualify the driver.
   - b. Certify the driver with a 1-time 3-month certificate.
   - c. Certify the driver for 1 year.
   - d. Certify the driver for 2 years.

82. A female driver reports for examination. Her current list of medications includes Effexor (venlafaxine) for what she reports was prescribed by her physician following her divorce last year. She noted that she is fine and really doesn't need it anymore. Her mannerism is fine and there is no apparent distress noted by the examiner. All other aspects of the examination are normal. The examiners best decision is to:
   - a. Temporarily disqualify the driver and request clearance for the medication and the condition from the prescribing provider.
   - b. Certify the driver for 1-year.
   - c. Certify the driver for 2 years.
   - d. Perform a Epworth questionnaire to determine if the medication was used as a sleep aide.

83. The driver reports a history of stroke 7 months earlier and presents a letter from his neurologist stating the he is cleared to return to work without restriction. The neurologist also submits office notes that indicate that the stroke was a thromboembolytic stroke, and that the driver suffers no deficits as a result in motor or cognitive abilities. All other aspects of the examination are within normal limits. The examination best certification decision is to:
   - a. Temporarily disqualify the driver
   - b. Request an EEG.
   - c. Certify the driver for 1 year.
   - d. Certify the driver for 2 years.

84. A driver reports that he must use hearing aides to drive. During the whisper test it is noted that even with the hearing aides, he is unable to detect a whispered voice at all in his right ear. In the left ear, he is however able to perceive a whispered voice at greater than 5 feet when tested. The examiners next step would be to:
   - a. Require the driver to apply for a hearing exemption.
   - b. Require the driver to have audiometric testing.
   - c. Certify the driver for 1 year, and mark "driving with the use of a hearing aide" on the certification status.
   - d. Certify the driver for 2 years, and mark "driving with the use of a hearing aide" on the certification status.

85. What is the waiting period for Benign Positional Vertigo (BPV)?
    a. 2 weeks.
    b. 1 month.
    c. 2 months.
    d. 3 months.

86. A driver who utilizes contact lenses to drive should be counseled to?
    a. To bring contact solution for overnight use.
    b. That they must have progressive lenses to be able to see both near and far.
    c. That they must bring a spare pair of glasses for use when they drive.
    d. That contacts may not be used while driving and they only may use traditional glasses to drive a CMV.

87. A driver marks in his history that he has recently been diagnosed with Obstructive Sleep Apnea or OSA and that he has begun using his CPAP a week ago without any difficulty. He provides copies of his sleep latency testing that was conducted a few weeks earlier that confirmed the diagnosis. The examiner should:
    a. Temporarily disqualify the driver.
    b. Request a CPAP compliance report.
    c. Certify the driver for 1 year.
    d. Certify the driver for 2 years.

88. During an examination of a male driver, the examiner identifies an inguinal hernia that is non reducible. Upon questioning, the driver reports that he has had this for quite some time (it was originally diagnosed a few years ago during a CDL exam), however he has noticed that it recently has become mildly painful with exertion but getting worse in the past week. The examiners best course of action would be to?
    a. Temporarily disqualify the driver and refer him for further medical evaluation.
    b. Have the driver perform a Functional Capacity Evaluation to determine if he is able to lift greater than 50 lbs.
    c. Certify the driver for 1 year.
    d. Certify the driver for 2 years.

89. What is the maximum certification period for Obstructive Sleep Apnea (OSA)?
    a. 6 months
    b. 12 months
    c. 18 months
    d. 24 months

90. A driver is missing all of his index finger in his right hand, but has a thumb and all of his other digits. He has a grip strength of 70 lbs "in right hand and exhibits in the CME's opinion to have good prehensal ability. The rest of the exam is within normal limits. The examiner should:
    a. Obtain a copy of the drivers driving record to determine if he has safely operated a CMV.
    b. Disqualify the driver.
    c. The driver may only be certified for a period of 1 year due to the missing digit.
    d. The driver may be certified for a period of 2 years.

91. When the examiner evaluates an audiometric test for hearing loss, what levels of testing (ANSI) are used to determine the drivers average hearing loss?
    a. 10 Htz, 20 Htz, and 50 Htz
    b. 50 Htz, 100 Htz, and 500 Htz
    c. 500 Ht, 1000 Htz and 2000 Htz
    d. 1000 Htz, 5000 Htz, and 10000 Htz

92. A 35-year old right handed female driver reports for a recertification. She reports in her history that she has recently been diagnosed with Carpal Tunnel Syndrome in her left wrist. Additionally, she reports using a brace at night, taking NSAIDS OTC PRN, and seeing her PCP and a physical therapist for treatment. She has no current restrictions from work. Her grip strength in her left hand is 4/5 and in her right hand is 5/5. The rest of her examination is unremarkable. The examiners next step should be to:
    a. Disqualify the driver and require her to apply for an SPE.
    b. Provide her with a temporary certificate for the duration of the physical therapy treatment to determine its success and obtain the opinion of her treating provider as to whether or not she can safely operate a CMV.
    c. Require that the driver see an Orthopedist for better evaluation of her CTS.
    d. Order a Nerve Conduction Test (NCV) to determine the extent of the driver's current compression.

93. A student at a local trucking school reports for a new certification. During the examination he reports he takes Zyprexa for the treatment of Schizophrenia. He presents a note from his psychologist stating that the condition is managed and he should be able to "drive". All other aspects of the examination are normal. The examiners best decision would be to:
    a. Request additional information from the psychologist relating to the side effects of Zyprexa.
    b. Require the driver to complete a Folsteins Mini Mental Health exam to determine is cognitive abilities.
    c. Certify the driver for 1 year because he suffers a mental disorder.
    d. Disqualify the driver.

94. A 56-year old male driver reports a history of "intermittent claudication". He is currently being treated by PCP and is due to see a vascular surgeon. He reports that his symptoms have worsened over the past year, and that he even has pain at rest. He takes a number of medications for his high blood pressure, for high cholesterol, and he takes ASA for pain PRN. During the exam, the examiner notices that the driver has a difficult time with ambulation, and the driver reports pain when he is sitting on the examination table. The examiners best decision would be to:
    a. Disqualify the driver.
    b. Provide a temporary certificate an allow the driver to see the vascular surgeon.
    c. Certify the driver for 1 year.
    d. Certify the driver for 2 years.

95. A 33-year old male driver reports a history of "Irritable Bowl Syndrome" or IBS. He is being treated with the use of diet and "Lomotil" and he reports he is well managed. He does not provide any release from his treating provider. The rest of his examination is unremarkable. The examiner best decision would be to:
    a. Request additional information from the treating provider.
    b. Certify the driver for 1 year.
    c. Certify the driver for 2 years.
    d. Disqualify the driver.

96. A 62-year old male driver reports for a recertification examination with a history of COPD. He reports that he smokes a pack and a half of cigarettes daily, and that he feels totally fine. The examination reveals positive findings during auscultation of the driver's lungs, he is slightly hypertensive, and over weight. During the examination he coughs frequently but it is non productive. Upon receiving medical records from the driver's pulmonologist, it confirms his diagnosis of COPD and it is revealed that he has suffered a "vasovagal syncope" resultant from coughing a few times over the past year. His pulmonary function test shows a FEV1 of 65, FVC of 61 and a FEV/FVC ration of 64. His ABG's were 68 and Pulse Ox was 93%. The examiner should:
    a. Disqualify the driver.
    b. Certify the driver for 6 months.
    c. Certify the driver for 1 year.
    d. Certify the driver for 2 years.

97. What is the minimum peripheral vision requirement of a driver?
    a. 90 degrees right and 90 degrees left.
    b. 80 degrees right and 80 degrees left.
    c. 70 degrees right and 70 degrees left.
    d. 60 degrees right and 60 degrees left.

98. During the evaluation of distance vision it is revealed that the driver is wearing contact lenses. His vision in his right eye with contact lenses is 20/20. His vision in his left eye is 20/60. The driver reports to the examiner that he uses one contact lens for near vision and one for far vision, but he carries a pair of glasses with him that have progressive lenses. Upon testing the drivers distance vision with his glasses only, he is 20/20 right and left. The examiners best decision would be to:
    a. Council the driver that he is not allowed to use his contact lenses when he drives, but he must only use his glasses, and certify the driver.
    b. Temporarily disqualify the driver and obtain the opinion of the driver's optometrist relating to the use of the contact lenses.
    c. Certify the driver with the use of his contact lenses or glasses as he meets the minimum vision requirements.
    d. Recommend that the driver have laser surgery to correct his vision.

99. What is the waiting period of a non-psychotic major depression, with no suicide attempt?
    a. There is no waiting period.
    b. 3 months
    c. 6 months
    d. 12 months

100. All of the following are symptoms of psychosis except:
   a. Euphoria
   b. Hallucinations
   c. Delusions
   d. Impaired insight

101. A driver has one ear canal completely plugged with wax but both ears pass the hearing standard. The medical exam is otherwise normal. What is the next step?
   a. Certify the driver for one year
   b. Certify the driver for 2 years
   c. Disqualify the driver until wax is removed.
   d. Temporarily qualify the driver and refer to a specialist

102. A driver complains of painless gradual loss of night vision, peripheral vision, and decreased color discrimination. Distance visual acuity has not changed. The most likely cause is:
   a. Macular degeneration
   b. Cataracts
   c. Glaucoma
   d. Retinopathy

103. A driver marks in his history that he has recently been diagnosed with Obstructive Sleep Apnea and that he began using his CPAP a week ago without any difficulty. He provides copies of his sleep latency testing that was conducted a few weeks earlier that confirmed the diagnosis. The examiner should:
   a. Temporarily disqualify the driver.
   b. Request a CPAP compliance report.
   c. Certify the driver for 1 year.
   d. Certify the driver for 2 years.

104. A driver reports that he uses hearing aides. During the whisper test it is noted that even when using the hearing aids, he is unable to detect a whispered voice in either ear. The driver fails audiometric testing without this hearing aids. What would be the next step?
   a. Disqualify the driver
   b. Counsel the driver regarding application for a hearing exemption.
   c. Require the driver to have open field audiometric testing prior to certification.
   d. Refer the driver to an ear specialist for evaluation prior to certification.

105. A driver must have a prescription for which of the following?
   a. Oxycodone
   b. Loratadine
   c. Certirizine
   d. Fexofenadine

106. An elderly driver is late by 1 hour to his appointment and says he gets lost easily. He struggled during his exam to remember his doctor's name and joked that it was due to his old age. His exam is otherwise normal. What is the next step?
   a. Qualify the driver for 1 year.
   b. Qualify the drive for 2 years.
   c. Disqualify the driver pending an evaluation from his PCP.
   d. Have the driver complete a MMSE exam.

107. A driver reports going in to the ER with chest pain 2 months ago. He states that he was advised to follow-up with his PCP, all tests were normal but he hasn't followed up with his doctor. His examination is within normal limits. What is the next step?
    a. Certify the driver for 2 years.
    b. Certify the driver for 1 year.
    c. Disqualify the driver and refer to his PCP.
    d. Disqualify the driver and refer to a cardiologist.

108. The driver has bilateral hand and arm tingling. There is a positive Tinel sign at the wrist. What should the ME order next?
    a. MRI of the head.
    b. CT of the cervical spine.
    c. Nerve conduction testing.
    d. TSH

109. While performing an abdominal exam you detect a bruit and a pulsing mass. What is the next step?
    a. Call emergency for transport to ER.
    b. Refer the driver immediately to his PCP.
    c. Disqualify the driver pending a CV evaluation.
    d. Counsel the driver regarding a need for evaluation of a possible AAA.

110. A driver weighs 500 lbs, eats only fast food and gets no exercise. His total cholesterol is 400 and his blood pressure is 138/88. Pulse is 99. The driver admits to not being faithful to using his statins and other medications as prescribed. The rest of his exam is unremarkable. What is the next step?
    a. Counsel the driver regarding low carb and low sodium diets.
    b. Caution the driver regarding non-compliance of medication and treatment plan.
    c. Disqualify the driver.
    d. Qualify the driver for one year.

111. You notice that the driver is wheezing and out of breath during the exam. What is the next step?
    a. PFT
    b. ABG
    c. Oximetry
    d. Refer to a pulmonologist.

112. A driver with COPD, hypertension and had a MI comes for re-certification. The results from the cardiologist were normal, however you notice the driver achieved 4.5 METs on the ETT. NO testing or evaluation was done for the COPD. What should the examiner do?
    a. Disqualify the driver
    b. Certify the driver for 3 months pending COPD evaluation.
    c. Certify the driver for 1 year.
    d. Disqualify the driver until it is determined that he meets the pulmonary guidelines for COPD.

113. What is the waiting period for surgical removal of a supratentorial tumor?
    a. 3 months
    b. 1 year
    c. 2 years
    d. 5 years

114. Which of the following does not have a 5 year waiting period?
    a. Stoke involving anterior or medial cerebral artery.
    b. Bacterial meningitis with early seizures.
    c. Stroke with risk for seizures.
    d. Moderate TBI without early seizures.

115. What is the waiting period and re-certification interval for a driver that has had a heart transplant?
    a. 3 months, and 1 year.
    b. 6 months, and 1 year.
    c. 1 year, and 6 months.
    d. 1 year, and 1 year.

116. Which of the following is a sign of "stable" angina?
    a. Pain at rest.
    b. Pain from exertion.
    c. Decreased response to medication.
    d. Pain of longer duration.

117. A driver with which of the following AAA's cannot be certified to drive?
    a. AAA size less than 4 cm and driver is asymptomatic.
    b. AAA size greater than 4 cm but less than 5 cm, asymptomatic with medical clearance.
    c. AAA size greater than 5 cm with CV specialist recommendation not to be repaired at this time.
    d. AAA is 3 cm and has increased less than .5 cm in the last 6 months.

118. A driver with a current medical certificate that does not expire for another year had an injury that interfered with his ability to drive. What is the next step?
    a. Driver can return to duty once healed.
    b. Driver can return to duty once released by the treating physician.
    c. Motor carrier may require the driver to return to the ME for evaluation.
    d. Driver must return to the ME for a medical examination.

119. A driver with diabetes reports partial loss of central vision, color discrimination, and obscured vision n the other vision fields. The most likely cause is?
    a. Macular degeneration
    b. Cataracts
    c. Glaucoma
    d. Retinopathy

120. What is the initial waiting period, and re-certification repeat ETT requirements for a driver with a history of MI?
    a. 2 month waiting period, and ETT annual
    b. 2 month waiting period, and ETT biennial
    c. 3 month waiting period, and ETT annual
    d. 3 month waiting period, and ETT biennial

ANSWERS TO PRACTICE TEST

Question 1: Correct answer is "d". An insulin dependant diabetic is disqualified until they obtain a diabetic exemption.

Question 2: Correct answer is "b". The driver is qualified to drive without restriction as long as he is able to perceive a whispered voice at 5 feet in 1 ear.

Question 3: Correct answer is "c". A driver may not use Chantix and drive a CMV and it must be confirmed that they are no longer taking the medication and that there are no effects from withdrawal, by the treating provider.

Question 4: Correct answer is "a". The driver has not completed the required 2 month waiting period but all other requirements for medical clearance and required testing have been met. The driver would be certified for 1 year at the completion of the remaining waiting period (2 weeks). The date of the certification would be from the date of the original examination.

Question 5: Correct answer is "b". The examiner would average the results from 500 Hz, 1000 Hz and 2000 Hz (required). This average is 38.33 in the Right and 43.33 in the Left ear. A driver must have an average hearing loss of less than or equal to 40 in the better ear. They do not have to meet this in both ears.

Question 6: Correct answer is "a". The driver is taking Antabuse which is used to treat alcohol addiction. This indicates that the driver currently suffers from a current clinical diagnosis of alcoholism.

Question 7: Correct answer is "c". Headache is not a typical symptom of congestive heart failure. Additional symptoms include wheezing, enlargement or prominent neck and facial veins, raised jugular venous pulse, bluish discoloration of face, presence of abnormal heart sounds, fatigue, weight gain and more.

Question 8: Correct answer is "a". A driver must exhibit a minimum peripheral vision of 70 degrees bilaterally.

Question 9: Correct answer is "b". The driver exhibits what may be considered a "Flat affect" which is seen in schizophrenia and in severe depression. The driver should be evaluated by a mental health expert to make a diagnosis prior to certification.

Question 10: Correct answer is "a". This is a best practice decision by the CME. If the CME determines the driver is capable is seeing his mirrors, and able to change lanes safely, he/she may be certified.

Question 11: Correct answer is "a". Use of marijuana is prohibited by Federal law while driving a CMV and trumps State law regarding this.

Question 12: Correct answer is "b". This is Stage 1 Htn, which is defined as 140 – 159/90 to 99.

Question 13: Correct answer is "d". Even though the driver has exceeded 10 years (required waiting period) it was not under medical supervision and the driver had discontinued his medication on his own. The waiting period would begin when the neurologist provides confirmation that the driver no longer requires medication (medical supervision).

Question 14 : Correct answer is "d". The driver who is diagnosed with OSA must have an annual sleep study (can be a sleep latency, wakefulness or Epworth test) and a CPAP compliance report. Since the exam is WNL the driver would be a limited risk and allowing enough time to provide this information to the examiner. If it meets minimum requirements or better, the driver may be certified for 1 year.

Question 15: Correct answer is "b". The driver must show at least 70% compliance.

Question 16: Correct answer is "a". Medical clearance is required for all mental disorders. Celexa is an SSRI or 2nd generation anti depressant and is ok for use with clearance also.

Question 17: Correct answer is "d". A driver with a history of TIA on anticoagulation therapy is automatically disqualified.

Question 18: Correct answer is "b". The driver must have a peripheral vision of 70 degrees bilaterally to certify to drive a CMV.

Question 19 ; Correct answer is "c". Blood oxygen saturation must be a minimum of 65% for the driver to certify.

Question 20: Correct answer is "a". Topomax is a medication that is used for seizure control. The examiner should confirm with the prescribing provider that the driver does not take it to control seizures, and they are capable of driving a CMV.

Question 21: Correct answer is "c". Certification for a driver with a vision exemption is annually and the driver must reapply for the exemption every 2 years.

Question 22: Correct answer is "d". The only two waiting periods that are 10 years are Epilepsy (no seizure and taken off of medication for 10 years), and Viral Encephalitis with early seizures.

Question 23: Correct answer is "c". Methadone is not allowed.

Question 24: Correct answer is "a". This is Stage 3 hypertension. The driver is disqualified until there blood pressure is less than 140/90 at which time they will have a maximum certification of 6 months for the rest of your career.

Question 25: Correct answer is "a". Because the driver has a history of hypertension (he is taking medication), and he had Stage 1 hypertension during his exam, he would be provided a 1-time, 3 month certificate in order to lower his blood pressure to an acceptable level during that time.

Question 26: Correct answer is "c". An A1c level of 10 equates to a blood glucose level of about 300 mg/dl. This is of little risk for a hypoglycemic event. You may certify the driver for only a period of 1 year if they are a diabetic. Also, metforman is not insulin.

Question 27: Correct answer is "d". A positive babinski reflex is indicative of abnormalities in the motor control pathways leading form the cerebral cortex and is widely used as a diagnostic aide in disorders of the central nervous system. The examiner should obtain clearance from a neurologist prior to reconsidering the driver for certification.

Question 28: Correct answer is "d". The driver's condition appears well controlled, they are under medical management for the condition and there is no history of incapacitation relating to their asthma. There is no advisory criteria limiting certification time and the driver may be certified for 2 years.

Question 29: Correct answer is "d". There are four required components of every examination, which are vision, hearing, blood pressure and UA. Ophthalmoscopic examination is not required but may be done if deemed necessary.

Question 30: Correct answer is "c". Byetta is an injectable non-insulin. Although it may require more frequent monitoring, the examiner may certify the driver for 1 year (shortened due to the treatment of diabetes).

Question 31: Correct answer is "d". The driver must have both the medical certification card and long form to apply for a vision exemption marked "certified for 1 year (required for all with a vision exemption), and "accompanied by a vision exemption" on each form. The exemption is good for two years even though the certification is limited to 1 year. It is the drivers responsibility to re apply and present the exemption at the time of the examination for each re certification.

Question 32: Correct answer is "b". You will need to obtain clearance from the treating provider to determine if the driver is able to drive a CMV. Areas of concern would be kidney function (obviously lacking), and if the driver suffers diabetes. If cleared other considerations would relate to how often the driver would need dialysis etc.

Question 33: Correct answer is "a". Following Coronary Artery Bi-pass Grafting (CABG), there is a 3-month waiting period. Since the driver is only at 8 weeks post-op, he would have to wait for about 4 more weeks until he can certify. Once he completes his waiting period he would be certified for 1 year from the date of the original examination.

Question 34: Correct answer is "a". Monovision (the use of one contact for close up vision and one for distance vision) is not allowed by the FMCSA. This would not require a specialist evaluation.

Question 35: Correct answer is "d". The driver is only able to take a sedative hypnotic at the lowest possible dose (must have a half-life of 5 hours) for a maximum duration of 2 weeks. The examiner should have confirmation from the prescribing provider that the driver is no longer taking the medication and clearance to drive prior to certifiction.

Question 36: Correct answer is "c". The driver has Stage 2 hypertension (160 to 179/100 to 109).

Question 37: Correct answer is "a". A driver who is diagnosed with Parkinson's is disqualified.

Question 38: Correct answer is "d". The driver is able to use hearing aides during the whisper test (and this should be marked on the form). A driver must only qualify in 1 ear to certify and there is no limitation of certification time.

Question 39: Correct answer is "b". The minimum acceptable values are 65%, 60% and 65% (FEV1, FVC, FEV1/FVC ration).

Question 40: Correct answer is "d". The abnormality in the UA is the level of blood in the urine, which is obviously a result of the driver's menstrual cycle. Without any other identified abnormality, the driver would be certified for 2 years.

Question 41: Correct answer is "d". Disqualify the driver because his angina is not stable.

Question 42: Correct answer is "c". Although you might be able to auscultate a bruit relating to a renal artery stenosis it would not be heard inferior to the sternal angle. Additionally, the palpable pulsation should further direct your thoughts to a AAA.

Question 43: Correct answer is "b". The driver may only be certified for a maximum of 6 months for the rest of his/her driving career.

Question 44: Correct answer is "a". The driver is not being treated for a mental condition such as anxiety or depression and he has clearance. He would be able to be certified for 2 years.

Question 45: Correct answer is "a". Council the driver concerning taking over the counter anti-histamines, and anti-tussives (both cause drowsiness and should not be taken while driving) about the 12-hour rule.

Question 46: Correct answer is "d". The driver suffered no seizures from the TBI, has completed the required waiting period (2 years), and has medical clearance. If the rest of the examination is unremarkable, the driver could be certified for 2 years.

Question 47: Correct answer is "c". The driver has a known cause for his episode, it only involved 1 event, no medication was required, and he has medical clearance. There is therefore no waiting period and the examiner may certify him for 2 years.

Question 48: Correct answer is "a". The driver is temporarily disqualified because he has not completed the mandatory waiting period for suicide attempt of 1 year. Once he has completed this, he may be certified for 1 year due to the continued treatment of depression (taking an SSRI). The certification is from the date of the originial examination.

Question 49: Correct answer is "c". The drivers hypothyroidism is well managed and he is asymptomatic. The driver may be certified for 2 years.

Question 50: Correct answer is "a". The driver suffers a chronic pain condition which may inhibit his ability to perform all essential functions associated with driving a CMV. He is also taking a narcotic medication. Both of these will need clearance from a treating provider prior to making a decision regarding certification.

Question 51: Correct answer is "c". A driver with A-Fib would require medical clearance. All drivers on anticoagulation therapy will require monthly INR readings. Normal values are 0.8 to 1.2, with values between 2 and 3 being acceptable. Because the driver has an irregular heartbeat, he must be certified for no greater than 1 year with medical clearance required.

Question 52: Correct answer is "d". The UA primarily evaluates kidney function and if the driver either suffers from diabetes or that their condition (diabetes) is well managed.

Question 53: Correct answer is "d". Despite admitting to having up to 14 beers on a weekend, he showed no clinical evidence in the examination to indicate he suffers from alcoholism, and his CAGE questionnaire score was only a 1 (a 2 or above would have required a temporary DQ until he has seen a SAP and provided a release).

Question 54: Correct answer is "c". A driver with TB is DQ'd until they have medical clearance, and have provided results of a chest X-ray, and pulmonary function test that meet or exceed minimum requirements to drive.

Question 55: Correct answer is "a". WPW Syndrome results in an arrhythmia that is often asymptomatic, but when symptomatic may be treated successfully medically or in some cases with an ablation. A successful ablation is assumed to "cure" the condition and post electrocardiography demonstrated a normal heart rate and rhythm, and the driver has the required medical clearance, has exceeded the required 3 months for the waiting period and due to his cardiac condition, his maximum certification is 1 year.

Question 56: Correct answer is "b". The driver has satisfied all requirements of the exemption, and an exemption is good for 2 years before the driver needs to reapply. Because they are treated for diabetes the maximum certification is for 1 year.

Question 57: Correct answer is "c". The driver shows signs of clubbing of the fingers and the examiner should request a specialists opinion regarding the driver condition.

Question 58: Correct answer is "d". The driver is significantly obese and has a medical history including diabetes and hypertension. This coupled with his admission of loud snoring would lead the examiner to be concerned that the driver suffers from obstructive sleep apnea. A sleep study would be the best choice for this driver.

Question 59: Correct answer is "d". The driver's condition and treatment do not appear to create any significant risk. There are no significant side effects that would interfere with safe operation of a CMV, and guidance does not limit the length of time that you can certify the driver.

Question 60: Correct answer is "b". A heavy menstrual cycle would not interfere with the certification process. With all other aspects of the driver's examination being unremarkable, the driver may be certified for a period of 2 years.

Question 61: Correct answer is "d". The waiting period for anyone who has attempted suicide is 1 year or 12 months.

Question 62: Correct answer is "a". Although the driver has clearance, he is required to have an annual ETT after 5 years. Even though his last ETT was acceptable (minimum acceptable is 6 mets) he will need to have one again before a final decision is made. Because his examination findings were unremarkable, and his previous ETT was well above minimum testing requirements, the best choice would be to provide a temporary certification with enough time to allow for him to complete required testing. If this is acceptable, he may be certified for 1 year.

Question 63: Correct answer is "c". The driver is disqualified because he is actively being treated for Psychosis.

Question 64: Correct answer is "d". Night sweats are not a symptom of core pulmonale. The others are. Additional symptoms include wheezing, chronic wet cough, enlargement or prominent neck and facial veins, raised jugular venous pulse, enlargement of the liver, bluish discoloration of the face, presence of abnormal heart sounds, and a bi-phasic response shown on an EKG due to hypertrophy.

Question 65: Correct answer is "b". The driver is required to have a pulmonary function test that would meet minimum requirements of an FEV1 of 65, FVC of 60 and FEV/FVC ration of 65.

Question 66: Correct answer is "b". The driver shows signs of central cynosis. There is a bluish discoloration of the tongue.

Question 67: Correct answer is "c". The only condition listed that would limit peripheral vision is glaucoma.

Question 68: Correct answer is "c". A driver with chronic tuberculosis that is taking streptomycin is disqualified.

Question 69: Correct answer is "b". The driver cannot perform all functions of his job despite being released for light duty.

Question 70: Correct answer is "d". The driver has a noticeable limitation in his left upper extremity. It should be determined if he has a "fixed deficit" and therefore would require a "Skill Performance Evaluation" or SPE.

Question 71: Correct answer is "d". Despite the driver having a pulse rate below 60, it is apparent during the exam that this relates to their high level of fitness and would not interfere with the safe operation of a CMV.

Question 72: Correct answer is "d". There are numerous variations of colorblindness, and the driver is only required to be able to distinguish between signal red, signal yellow and signal green.

Question 73: Correct answer is "a". The driver is truly not under any active treatment for their alcoholism, and has exhibited no evidence of currently suffering an active case of alcoholism. They would be certified for a period of 1 year due to the fact they are treated for hypertension.

Question 74: Correct answer is "c". Aricept is a medication that is used in the treatment of Alzheimer's disease. Any dementia, including that associated with Alzheimer's, is disqualifying. Once confirmed, the driver would be permanently disqualified.

Question 75: Correct answer is "a". There is a 1-week waiting period for angioplasty or Percutaneous Coronary Intervention (PCI).

Question 76: Correct answer is "d". The UA is used to determine kidney function (specific gravity, protein and blood), and diabetes (specific gravity and sugar).

Question 77: Correct answer is "b". All others meet the FMCSA definition of a driver who has a clinical case of epilepsy.

Question 78: Correct answer is "a". The driver has met all requirements post PCI and the initial certification must be for 3 to 6 months. Following this, as long as they have met their certification requirements (medical clearance, ETT biannual), they may be certified for a period of 1 year.

Question 79: Correct answer is "d". Individuals who suffer sickle cell anemia used to have a shortened life expectancy (average age 42 years), but with recent advances in treatment, their life expectancy is now into the 80's. They do however have a tendency to suffer a number of crises during their life, and they must be managed medically throughout their life. They have a greater chance for infection, episodes of anemia and stroke. It would therefore be prudent to certify them for 1 year instead of 2 in order to monitor their condition more closely.

Question 80: Correct answer is "d". The driver may be provided only 1 3-month temporary certificate during a 12-month period. Because he did not responsibly follow up with his provider or providing the examiner with a confirmed acceptable blood pressure, he would be disqualified until these requirements are met.

Question 81: Correct answer is "c". The driver suffers from Stage 1 hypertension. Since this is the first time detected, meaning that there is no previous history of hypertension, the driver may be certified for 1 year. If there was a history, or if the driver suffered from Stage 2 hypertension, he would have been issued a 1-time, 3-month certificate to allow him to obtain a blood pressure below 140/90.

Question 82: Correct answer is "a". The driver suffers from a mental disorder (depression) and even though it appears to be well managed, it is required that the examiner receive medical clearance from the treating provider prior to certification.

Question 83: Correct answer is "a". The driver is temporarily disqualified because they have not met the required 1 year waiting period.

Question 84: Correct answer is "d". The driver meets minimum requirements for driving with the use of a hearing aide. There is no limitation in certification time therefore the driver may be certified for 2 years. The examiner must also mark the certification status as "driving with the use of hearing aides".

Question 85: Correct answer is "c". The waiting period for BPV is 2 months.

Question 86: Correct answer is "c". They must bring a spare pair of glasses.

Question 87: Correct answer is "a". The driver has not met the minimum 1-month waiting period for use of a CPAP. Once complete they may be certified for 1 year.

Question 88: Correct answer is "a". This is due to the fact that the hernia is non reducible and symptomatic, and the pain is worsening.

Question 89: Correct answer is "b". The maximum certification time for a driver with OSA is 12 months or 1 year.

Question 90: Correct answer is "d". Because the driver exhibits a strong grip strength and has good prehensal ability the CME driver should be certified for 2 years.

Question 91: Correct answer is "c". The driver may not have greater than 40db of hearing loss in the better ear as measured at 500 Htz, 1000 Htz and 2000 Htz.

Question 92: Correct answer is "b". The best answer of the available choices would be to provide her with a temporary certificate and reevaluate. An SPE is not required because CTS is not a "Fixed Deficit".

Question 93: Correct answer is "d". Scizophrenia is a permanent psychiatric disorder and is always a disqualifying condition.

Question 94: Correct answer is "a". A driver who suffers intermittent claudication who suffers pain at rest must be disqualified.

Question 95: Correct answer is "c". The condition is well managed and there is no guidance that would shorten his certification time. He may be certified for 2 years.

Question 96: Correct answer is "a". The driver suffers from COPD with cough syncope. He is automatically disqualified.

Question 97: Correct answer is "c". The driver must exhibit a minimum of 70 degrees of peripheral vision both right and left.

Question 98: Correct answer is "a". A driver is not allowed to use two different contact lenses, one for near vision, and one for far vision.

Question 99: Correct answer is "c". The waiting period is 6 months.

Question 100: Correct answer is "a". Euphoria is not a symptom of psychosis.

Question 101: Correct answer is "c". The ME must view the tympanic membrane and auditory canal prior to certification.

Question 102: Correct answer is "C" Intraocular pressure causes progressive atrophy of nerve cells. Symptoms include redirection of visual attention, and decreased peripheral, night vision, and color discrimination for certain colors.

Question 103: Correct answer is "a". There is a waiting period of 1-month once a CPAP is prescribed, prior to the driver returning to work.

Question 104: Correct answer is "c". Open field testing is used to perform audiometric testing prior to certification. Refer the driver for testing prior to certification. In this way, the driver wearing hearing aids may meet the audiometric standard and not need a hearing exemption.

Question 105: Correct answeer is "a". Drivers must have a prescription for a narcotic (Oxycodone). The others are over the counter medications.

Question 106: Correct answer is "d. The MMSE exam result may indicate that a referral to a mental health specialist is required.

Question 107: Correct answer is "c". When a referral has been made from a healthcare provider the ME should refer to the PCP for evaluation prior to certification.

Question 108: Correct answer is "c". This driver may have nerve interference best determined by a nerve conduction test.

Question 109: Correct answer is "a". Upon detection of a AAA with high risk of rupture, the ME should provide or initiate immediate emergency care.

Question 110: Correct answer is "b". ME's should discuss non-compliance of treatment plan and medication use with the driver.

Question 111: Correct answer is "d". Drivers that exhibit wheezing and/or are out of breath during the exam should have a pulmonary evaluation prior to certification.

Question 112: Correct answer is "a". Drivers must exceed 6 METs on an ETT to be qualified to drive.

Question 113: Correct answer is "c". The waiting period for removal of a supratentorial tumor is two years.

Question 114: Correct answer is "d". Moderate TBI without early seizures has a waiting period of 2 years.

Question 115: Correct answer is "c". A driver who has had a heart transplant must wait one year if asymptomatic, tolerates medication, has CV clearance no signs of rejection and if they meet all other CV requirements he/she may be certified for a period of 6 months.

Question 116: Correct answer is "b". Stable angina includes pain with exertion, emotion, extremes in weather and sexual activity.

Question 117: Correct answer is "c". Regardless for recommendations for no repair, AAA's over 5 cm are disqualifying.

Question 118: Correct answer is "d". When a driver returns from an illness or injury that interferes with his/her driving ability, the driver must undergo a medical examination even if the medical examiner's certificate has not expired.

Question 119: Correct answer is "d". Diabetes is the most common cause of retinopathy. Partial loss of central and obscured vision in other fields is possible. Color discrimination also may be affected.

Question 120: Correct answer is "b". Drivers who are post MI have a 2 month waiting period, and after the initial certification bust have an ETT every two years.

NOTES

_____

_____

_____

_____

_____

_____

_____

_____

_____

_____

_____

_____

NOTES

NOTES

Made in the USA
Middletown, DE
03 September 2023

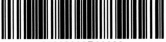